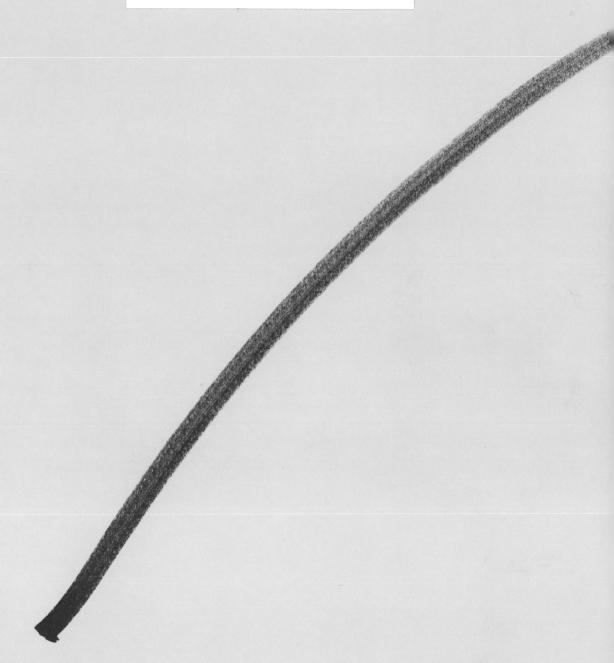

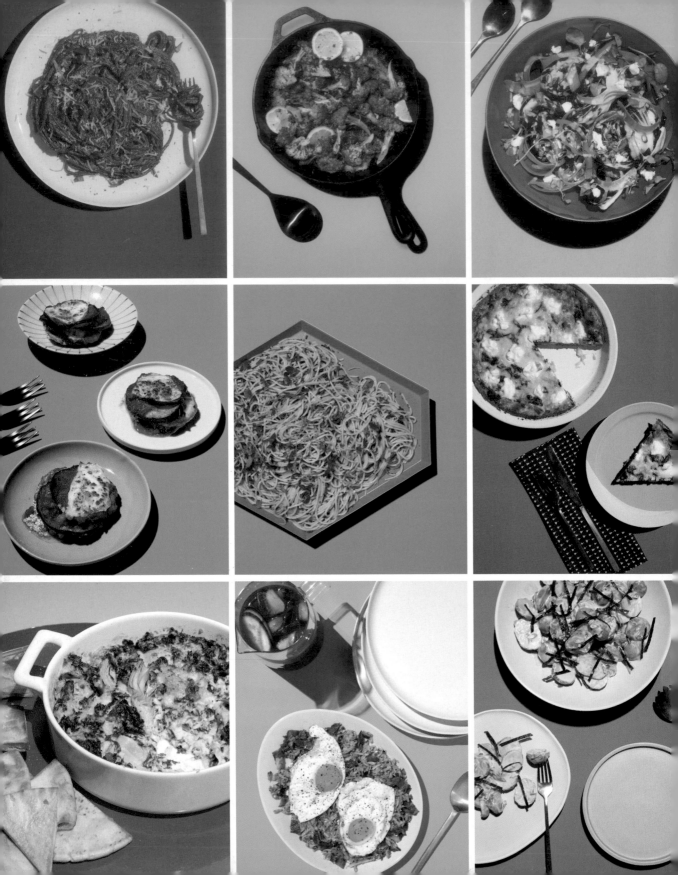

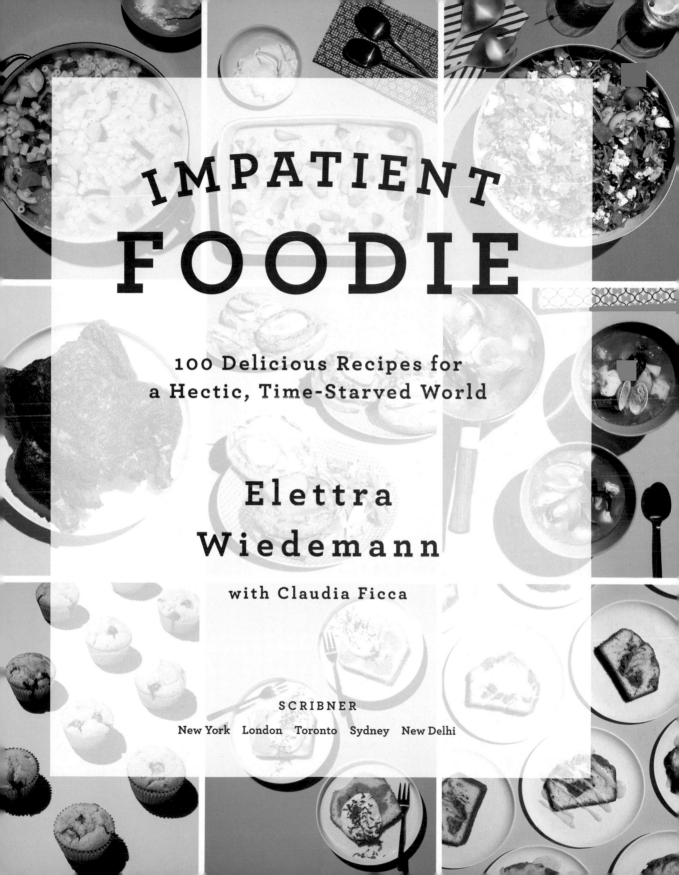

IMPATIENT
FOODIE

100 Delicious Recipes for
a Hectic, Time-Starved World

Elettra
Wiedemann

with Claudia Ficca

SCRIBNER

New York London Toronto Sydney New Delhi

SCRIBNER
An Imprint of Simon & Schuster, Inc.
1230 Avenue of the Americas
New York, NY 10020

First Scribner hardcover edition June 2017

SCRIBNER and design are registered trademarks of The Gale Group, Inc.,
used under license by Simon & Schuster, Inc., the publisher of this work.

For information about special discounts for bulk purchases,
please contact Simon & Schuster Special Sales at 1-866-506-1949
or business@simonandschuster.com.

The Simon & Schuster Speakers Bureau can bring authors to your live event.
For more information or to book an event, contact the Simon & Schuster Speakers Bureau
at 1-866-248-3049 or visit our website at www.simonspeakers.com.

Interior design by Erich Hobbing

Manufactured in the United States of America

1 3 5 7 9 10 8 6 4 2

Library of Congress Cataloging-in-Publication Data is available.

ISBN 978-1-5011-2891-2
ISBN 978-1-5011-2893-6 (ebook)

This book is dedicated to my grandad,
who always inspired me to think harder, dream bigger,
and taught me how to cook the perfect salmon fillet in just ten minutes
with three ingredients when I was nine years old,
thus igniting my *Impatient Foodie* fire.

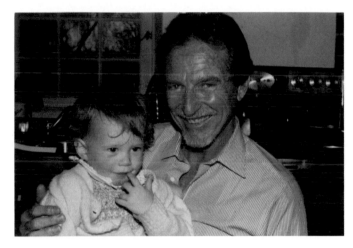

Fred "Grandad/Afi" Wiedemann (1923–2017)

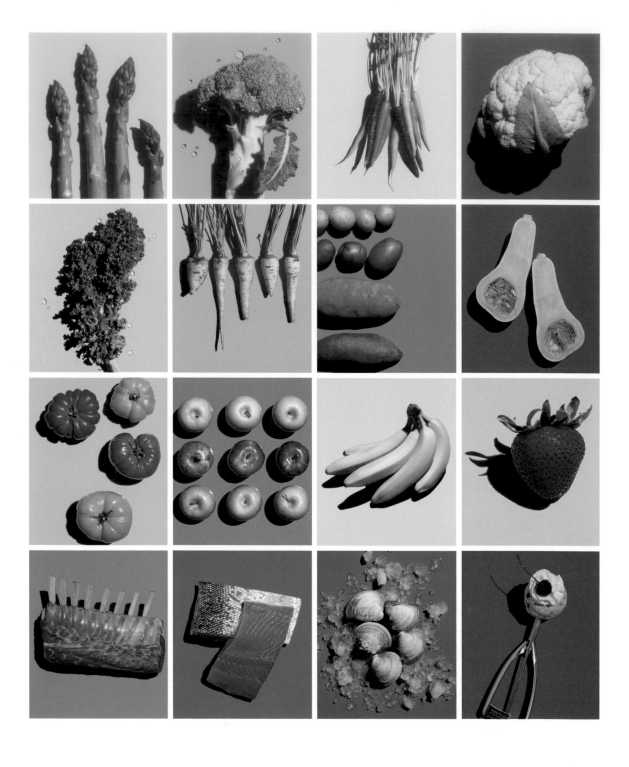

TABLE OF CONTENTS

CHICKEN, MEAT, FISH

FRUITS

THROW 'EM TOGETHER DESSERTS

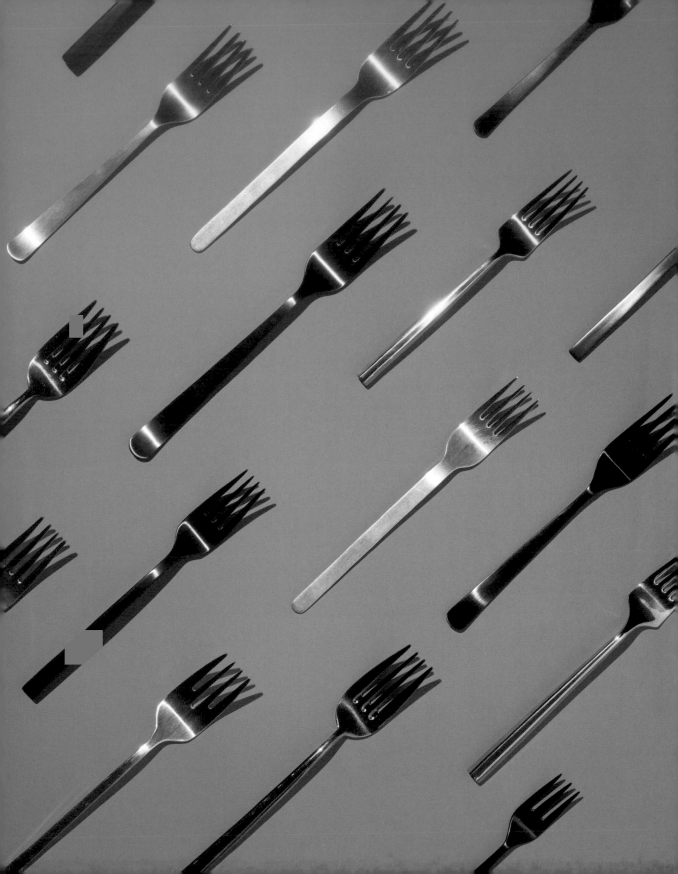

INTRODUCTION

Ten years ago if you had told me I'd be a food blogger and cookbook author, I would have chuckled and patted you on the head. Until I was about twenty-seven, the only relationship I had with food was what I cooked for myself to make sure I could fit into sample sizes for modeling work. I had always pretty much subsisted on pasta (tortellini!), but that stopped working when it came to fitting into size 2 clothes. But the financial upside of being unnaturally thin at almost six feet tall was a good enough incentive for me to reel in my love for pasta and teach myself how to eat more cleanly. I focused on integrating more vegetables into my diet, but also not starving myself because, to paraphrase the Hulk, "you wouldn't like me when I am hungry." After a few years of experimenting, I got to a place where I could cook myself very healthy meals that provided the same satisfaction as a bowl of my weakness—tortellini drowned in pesto and olive oil.

Learning to cook and feed myself in a new way was the unwitting first step on my road to foodie-ism. The second one came a few years into modeling, when I experienced what I call my "Quarter-Life Crisis." I suddenly freaked and decided that disappearing into Africa was the only way to clear my head. I volunteered at Oria and Iain Douglas-Hamilton's Save the Elephants camp in the Samburu National Reserve. There I was put in charge of stocking the camp's food supply. Within days, I was flabbergasted (and slightly disgusted, to be perfectly frank) when I realized the incredible quantity of food that humans consume. I remember one morning in particular, while I was counting the supplies, when I thought, "What the hell, we're out of that already?! God, if fifteen people are going through this in a week, imagine what a city like New York goes through, or London, or Beijing!" Still today, when I try to imagine that quantity of food, it is so large that I can't. (Don't even get me started on the amount of food waste—that just makes me want to cry.)

A few years later, I got accepted to the London School of Economics for grad school. I didn't feel some major calling toward academia, mostly I applied there on a whim. Hey, if I got accepted into the biomedicine program, wouldn't that be impressive?! Oh shit, I got accepted. No one was more surprised than me. In addition to my requirement courses, I took classes in environmental politics and cultural theory. There was zero strategy or vision in my curriculum choices beyond interest, curiosity, and recommendations from friends. But my random approach to classes really bit me in the ass when it came time to propose my dissertation topic: What connects public health, environment, and cultural phenomena? After weeks of wracking my brain, the answer became clear: food. I wrote my dissertation on the future of feeding urban populations with a particular focus on a biotechnology proposal known as vertical farming. I can feel your eyes glazing over as you read that, so I'll just say it was through researching that I came to realize that food is much more than just what's on my plate. It connected me right to all the large, complex, inertia-inducing issues that kept me awake at night, like climate change, water (or lack thereof), the state of the oceans, human rights, animal rights, and beyond.

But in spite of knowing all I knew, I was IMPATIENT.

Every time I stood in front of my supermarket's egg aisle, I was filled with befuddlement, frustration, and confusion—this cocktail of feelings inspired me to start *Impatient Foodie*. What I want is simple: eggs that are healthy for me and come from a healthy, happy chicken. Yet I find myself reading the damn cartons for at least ten to fifteen minutes, weighing my options with an inner monologue that goes something like: "These eggs are organic, but not certified humane. Those are certified humane, but not organic. This carton says their eggs are organic and the chickens were cage-free, but no humane certification. These are organic and have that non-GMO butterfly seal. . . . Wait, how does that make sense? Isn't that redundant? Whatever, don't get sidetracked—FOCUS. These just have cute chicken cartoons on the carton with lots of great words and promises, but no official seals of any kind. But, still the cartoons have to mean something, right?! No one could be that cynical or dishonest . . . could they?" Time ticks by, my shopping list doesn't get any shorter, and at some point I throw my hands up in frustration and just toss whatever egg carton into

the cart. Then I move on to the next thing on my list, which inevitably involves its own set of mind-bending questions and moral quandaries. My close friends and family stopped shopping with me a long time ago.

And to be totally honest—and at the risk of hurting what I am trying to help here—my frustration doesn't come to an end when I go to the farmers' market. Sure, I might spend substantially less time and energy fretting over sourcing, but I'm pushing my way through hundreds (if not thousands) of other customers, stopping by multiple cash-only (why?!) stalls, lugging bags to and fro, and dodging the usual NYC characters, hawkers, and maybe even some singing Hare Krishna. The chaos and lack of convenience grates on my patience. If I've had a bad day or the weather isn't within my Goldilocks range, I might skip the farmers' market all together and use a food delivery app.

But you know what—except for a few saints out there—aren't you at least a little bit like me, deep down?

The Slow Food movement and its thought leaders—like Michael Pollan, Mark Bittman, Alice Waters, and Joan Gussow—have shown how the ripple effects of what we eat go wide: Food isn't just about personal health, it affects the rights and protection of farm workers; the quality of soil, water, fossil fuel usage, carbon release, and sequestration; animal rights; the health of our oceans, and more. And who doesn't want to be part of that? I know that I do. I want to have a positive role in helping to reshape the food system to be healthier, more sustainable, more transparent, more humane, and more democratic for all. I totally understand and see how the food choices I make affect not only my health, but my future children's health, and the planet's health.

But it's also true that when I stand in front of the suffocating amount of options at my local market's egg aisle, or I get bulldozed way too many times at the farmers' market, I also just want to lie down in my bed, claim ignorance, and order my meals on a food delivery app. What it comes down to is that I want to participate in food activism, but I am also impatient, overworked, time strapped, tired, I often feel stretched very thin . . . and sometimes—I'll admit—I am lazy as hell.

For a long time, I felt alone and ashamed of this duality in me: How can someone want to participate in something they know is important but also feel like the whole "think globally, shop locally!" thing can be a real time-sucking drag? I felt doubly ashamed because I studied these very issues at the London School of Economics, so I could not claim ignorance or lack of understanding. And while I wish SO VERY HARD that my knowledge would override my impatience, that is sadly not the case all the time. And the more I tried to silence or squash my impatient side, with rationales like "but it's good for you and good for the planet!" the more the impatient voice would rise. But I kept quiet about my inner eye-rolling because everything I read and heard was more in the vein of, "Isn't the farmers' market so lovely?! Let's listen to this guy talk about his small-batch pickling technique for forty-five minutes! Aren't these sweet, small-batch jams so incredible?! Let's bake them in a homemade pie, made from scratch. Or, better yet, let's spread the jam on

homemade sourdough bread that takes fifteen hours to make! Don't you just love spending your entire day dealing with or talking about food?" Hell NO. Oh, erm—sorry, I mean, no I don't really enjoy that so much, but I am so glad you do! (That's a more mature response, right?)

There was also a fight between the slow-food recipes I was finding and the busy life I was constrained by. I dreamed of making that amazing slow-braised dinner I saw on the *Bon Appétit* website, but by the time I got home I only had the time and energy to eat something more along the lines of what I could order for takeout on my phone. I started self-flagellating because I felt like a total "foodie fraud." The idea of laboring over anything in the kitchen for more than one hour (or, really, thirty minutes, pretty please?) is plainly unrealistic for me.

If you feel the same way, this cookbook is for you. The recipes herein are all inspired by the simple philosophy: Good, thoughtful, healthy meals need to be easier, faster, and more fun.

My goal with *Impatient Foodie* is three-fold: 1) To serve up *Bon Appétit*–style meals in *Buzz-Feed* time. 2) To encourage people to shop at farmers' markets whenever possible, to cook at home, and to engage with their food in a time when home cooking is on a downward trend across the nation. I think this is the first step toward awakening understanding of the larger issues at stake; I know it has been for me. 3) To have *Impatient Foodie* be part of an honest conversation between the leaders of the Slow Food movement and those of us living in cities, doing our best to participate, but feeling a little, well, stretched. I know it's not ideal to say that people are impatient, addicted to convenience, and lazy: Just don't be impatient! Don't be lazy! I think that will change someone's shopping habits for a couple days, maybe a few weeks, but certainly not forever. Eventually, all those realities come cascading back in, no matter how much we lament or resist or despise them. Basically what I have to say is this: Enough with the aspiration!!!! In order to change the food system, let's look at where we really are, what human nature really is, how people are trying and failing, and figure out how can we meet in the middle to work toward a common goal—a sustainable, more transparent, more equitable food system.

This cookbook has been designed with time constraints and impatience in mind. To make the book extra user friendly, we based our recipes around ingredients. For example, did you get inspired to buy beets at the farmers' market only to realize you have zero idea what to do with them when you got home? We've got your back with four beet-centric suggestions for you that include an appetizer, a main, a side, and even a dessert. Or maybe you have a mini mountain of herbs slowly, sadly wilting in your fridge after you used just four leaves as a garnish?

We've been there too, and have a number of suggestions for how to use them ranging from soup to dessert. There are a total of twenty-one main ingredients in here with nearly 100 recipe suggestions for impatient cocktails, appetizers, mains, sides, and desserts that are delicious and that you'll be proud to serve and share.

For the record, I know this is a not "perfect" cookbook. I am sure my luminaries like Pollan, Bittman, Waters, or Gussow would not be impressed by some of my choices, like the use of store-bought cake mixes to streamline baking (it's just too much otherwise). Sometimes coordinating the recipes to only seasonal ingredients was impossible at maximum, and totally maddening at minimum. But you know what—I'M TRYING. And also, recipes are always flexible! If you can't find a certain ingredient at your market, skip it! Or sub in something else that's there that you know will be yummy. Cooking is all about your own personal flair.

In a nutshell, *Impatient Foodie* is my attempt to reconcile my earnestness and desire to do my part with my extreme impatience (and, let's face it, occasional laziness). I know that I am not alone.

NOTES ON HOW TO READ A RECIPE

Mise en place Do you hate doing the dishes? Me too—it's such a bore! When I was forced to tackle a sinkful as a kid, I would pretend that I was on TV hosting a dishwashing show to entertain myself while I worked through it. Unfortunately, dirty dishes are an inevitable part of the cooking process. But there is a way to minimize chaos in the kitchen: the mise en place. Translated roughly from French to English this means, "get your ducks in a row before you start cooking." In other words, do all your measuring, chopping, slicing, grating, or whatevering before you actually start to cook. What to prepare for your mise en place will be clear from the ingredients section of all the recipes. You'll see that the ingredients section indicates the quantities and also preparation of any given ingredient. For example:

1 eggplant, washed and halved
1 lemon, zested and juiced
2 tablespoons honey

I know the mise en place may sound like an extra step, but really it's not—you're going to be chopping or measuring all the stuff anyway. But this way you're just doing the prep as the first step. I promise that it will really streamline the whole cooking process for you. And—SUPER BONUS!—no more kitchen crises: those pan-icked, pull-your-hair-out moments when food is practically on fire in the pan, you're trying to focus on chopping something, you're pulling out plates and utensils left and right to keep things in order, you suddenly realize that you forgot to add something to the pan, and—AHHHH!!—the smoke alarm just went off! Cut to you throwing up your hands in frustration, screaming profane words, dumping it all in the trash, and calling in food (I feel you, I've been there).

Ingredients list We have also listed our ingredients in the order of use to help keep the cooking process and steps extra crystal clear. So if you're cooking a pasta dish, you might not see it listed as the first ingredient if it's not being used first.

In some recipes you'll be using a given ingredient more than once—say, maybe at the beginning and again at the end—but they won't be listed twice in the ingredients list, so it is important to read all the instructions first to familiarize yourself with the steps and know if an ingredient will be divided.

Similarly, in cases where there is an ingredient listed without a quantity (for example just "extra virgin olive oil" with no cup, tablespoon, or teaspoon measure), it means that you'll be using it in several places throughout the recipe and specific quantities or directions will be listed in the instructions. Furthermore, the instructions assume that you have already done the prep as stated in the ingredients list. So if you read an instruction that says "add asparagus to the pot" you have to make sure those asparagus stalks have been prepped properly. We also assumed you have washed all your fruits and vegetables before getting started.

Water Water is never listed in the ingredients list, but if you need to use it we will specify quantities in the instructions.

Heat Also, pretty please follow the instructions on the heat level. If you read an instruction that says, "cook over medium-low heat" and think to yourself, "HA! I am going to quicken this up by cooking it on high heat. I am a genius!" (again, I've been there), please don't do that. We spent hundreds of hours testing out these recipes multiple times. If our instructions say to cook something over a certain heat, it's not to slow you down—I wouldn't do that to you.

Salt We used kosher salt in the development of all these recipes. Why does that matter? Well, all salt is salty (obviously), but salt particles can be different sizes. For example, grains of table salt are a lot finer than grains of kosher salt. So if a recipe calls for 1 teaspoon kosher salt and you use 1 teaspoon of table salt, you risk oversalting your dish (and there's no easy recovery from oversalting something). If you can, I recommend getting a big box of kosher salt and storing it in your pantry (We use Morton's kosher salt). Also, we occasionally use Maldon salt (big

sea salt flakes), but we're careful to make the distinction in recipes where it is used.

Stock We used store-bought organic chicken, vegetable, and fish stocks and I am unapologetic about that. Making stock from scratch is an impatient foodie's nightmare. I mean, if you can do it and you want to do it, by all means—stock your heart out! Homemade stock is undoubtedly far more delicious than what you can buy at the store. However, in my experience it's hours and endless hours of messy work, not to mention a lot of cleanup. The good news? Because bone broths are the new green juice, I am seeing a lot of frozen bone broths available at farmers' markets these days (some vendors hide their bone broths in coolers under the tables, so you might have to ask). Any kind of meat-based stocks or bone broths can be used interchangeably for the purposes of all of these recipes.

Doubling a recipe Oh, and one more thing: Most of the recipes in this book serve 4 to 6 people. If you're planning a dinner party and need to cook for 8 to 12 people, you can double any recipe to get the same results. But I highly recommend that you use a pencil to write in the doubled quantities before you get started on your mise en place or start cooking. I can't tell you how many times I have just ploughed into a recipe in an impatient haste, only to be halfway through cooking or baking it and realize that I doubled only half of the ingredients and forgot about the rest: *No bueno* and easily avoidable with the help of a pencil.

A WORD ON IMPATIENCE AND DESSERTS

You won't find me baking that much, because most baking requires a lot of patience. I read recipes and think, "Wait. I have to wait how long to let this rise? Forget it." And you can't blast cookies at higher heat because they'll just get burnt to a sad, not tasty, crisp. That being said, a home-baked anything is awesome and a sure way to impress (yourself, if no one else). In this cookbook, we've provided many dessert ideas to help get you baking, all of which are impatient friendly. The desserts made from scratch have minimal ingredients; the cake, muffin, and scone recipes use store-bought mixes to streamline the process and spare you from the time and mess of measuring out ingredients like flour, baking soda, baking powder, etc. And there are a few options that are even less work than that: no-bake desserts that simply involve assembling store-bought ingredients in "Throw 'Em Together Desserts." Whatever the occasion for a sweet treat and however impatient you're feeling, we've got your back.

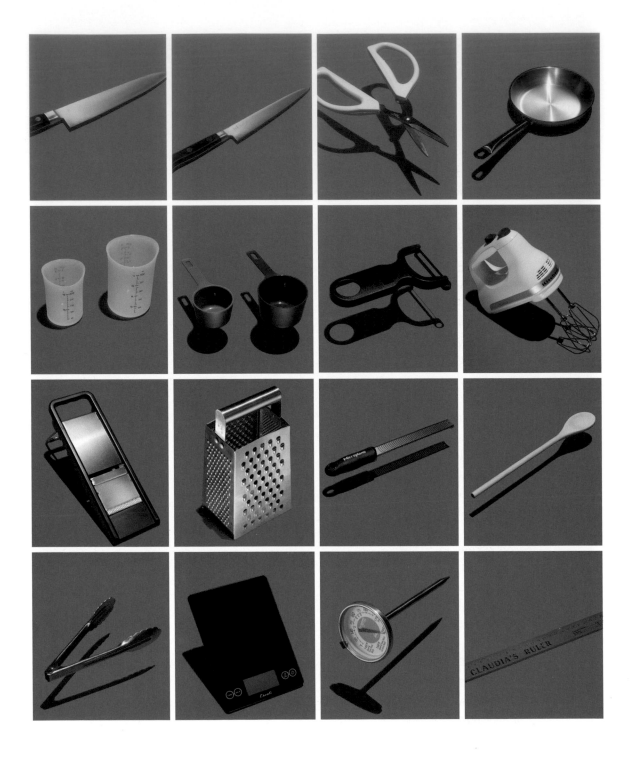

IMPATIENT FOODIE
KITCHEN FAVORITES

Many cookbooks have a section devoted to "Pantry Essentials" or "The Perfect Pantry" with a long list of specialty spices that always discourages me for some reason. In the past, I have unquestioningly followed these kinds of instructions from certain-people-who-shall-remain-nameless only to be left with spices in my pantry that go unused (or unopened) for years. For example, I've had a large container of cumin in my pantry now for about three years, because I don't really like it and never use it. In fact, I tend to veer away from recipes that have a lot of cumin. So I decided to skip such a list and tell you that I am a big believer in accruing and collecting spices according to your own tastes and cooking habits over time. I could have saved myself that cash to use toward various tools that really made my cooking life easier, and helped me build my confidence (and speed) in the kitchen.

The following kitchen items have made my life easier and my cooking go faster. These are also the tools we repeatedly use in this cookbook. Most of this stuff is not expensive, or can be found at a lower price point.

1) A really sharp chef's knife—Consider this your best friend in the kitchen. Splurging on a good chef's knife will make any chopping, cutting, or mincing much faster and easier.

2) Kitchen shears—These are an impatient foodie's best friend when it comes to doing things quickly, like snipping herbs or cutting the backbone out of a chicken. They are also helpful in opening food packaging and more.

3) A large, thick cutting board—Pro tip: Place an unfolded, moist paper towel underneath your cutting board to help it stay in place while you cut on it.

4) Ovenproof and dishwasher-safe pots and pans—I find cast iron skillets to be completely overrated, except for the fact that they transfer easily from stovetop to oven. Luckily for all of us, there are a lot of great brands that make ovenproof pots and pans that are light and can be washed in the dishwasher. I highly recommend NOT getting pots and pans coated with nonstick coating, which can be toxic if overheated (obviously a risk if you're cooking/baking at high temperatures). If you have limited space or budget, these are my workhorses:

- A large (11- to 12-inch) sauté pan or skillet
- A large pot for boiling water and making soups
- A couple of saucepans with lids (these come in multiple sizes, so get what

makes sense for your household and how many people you are cooking for)

- A standard roasting pan (17 x 13 x 3 inches)

5) Baking pans—Here are the basics:

- At least two 15 x 10-inch baking sheets (useful for soooo many things, from split roast chicken to cookies)
- Two 9-inch round cake pans
- A standard 12-cup muffin tin (each cup is 2½ inches across and 1¼ inches deep)
- A standard loaf pan (9 x 5 x 3 inches)

6) A colander—This is a must for straining pasta and just about anything else.

7) Nonreactive metal bowls of varying sizes—I didn't consider these a kitchen essential until I took some cooking classes—they are a game changer and make cooking life much easier. They are light, stackable, incredibly easy to wash or rinse out, unbreakable, and cheap.

8) Measuring cups and measuring spoons—Obviously important to, you know, measure things. There are two kinds of measuring cups: Those that measure dry ingredients, like flour and sugar, and a liquid measuring cup, which will have measurements for fluid ounces on the side.

- Measuring shot glass—Take the stress and guesswork out of converting cocktail recipes from ounces into tablespoons with this little guy.

9) A peeler—Easily and quickly peel vegetables and fruits. You can also use a peeler to ribbon vegetables like asparagus and carrots (see pages 10 and 33).

10) Handheld electric mixer—An electric mixer is the lazy/impatient foodie's whisk. Just hold it steady and let the mixer do the work. Especially helpful when making whipped cream.

11) Food processor—For years I resisted getting a food processor for no reason at all. Once I got one it was immediately clear that I had been a stubborn idiot. Food processors are the jam—I hug mine sometimes. I recommend getting a 12-cup food processor, if you have the storage space for it. I also had a smaller one when I was in my small NYC apartment with limited shelf space, and it was still a great tool to have.

12) A blender or immersion blender—If you have to choose between buying a food processor or blender for budget reasons, I personally would get the food processor. But a powerful blender is great for more liquid-based pureeing, like making smoothies. If you don't enjoy smoothies but you love soups, then I would suggest getting an immersion blender, which means you can puree right in the pot you are cooking the soup in and not transfer hot liquid into a blender.

13) Mandoline—Rather than enduring the painstaking process of thinly slicing whatever ingredient with a knife, you can easily, quickly, and perfectly slice on a mandoline.

14) Kevlar gloves—These will help to save your fingers from getting accidentally sliced by the mandoline.

15) Box grater—If you love freshly grated cheese, then a box grater is your best

friend. Also useful for other recipes that you'll find in this cookbook.

16) Rasp-style zester—I used to think a rasp-style zester was unnecessary if you owned a box grater, but I was wrong. A box grater just doesn't do the same job of finely zesting stuff like lemons, limes, oranges, fresh ginger, garlic, etc.

17) Wooden spoons—These are essential because wooden spoons don't transfer heat to your hand while cooking over a boiling pot of water or in a skillet.

18) Heat resistant silicone spatulas—Like wooden spoons, heat resistant silicone spatulas won't transfer heat to your hands, but they are more manipulatable, which comes in handy when dealing with batters/baking.

19) Metal tongs—You can use a wooden spoon, spatula, or even a fork to help pull hot pasta out of a boiling pot of water, or turn over sizzling bacon, but metal tongs make those tasks faster and easier.

20) Kitchen scale—I survived without a kitchen scale for quite a while and did just fine. But when I finally bought one for myself, I found that it really did help to minimize the stress of converting recipes I found listed in grams, ounces, pounds rather than cups, tablespoons, and teaspoons. Sometimes in this book you'll see things measured in pounds, because cups or tablespoon measurements would not have been accurate.

21) Instant-read thermometer—The days of hacking into your beautiful chicken or fillet of fish to see if they're cooked are over with the help of a handy, instant-read meat thermometer.

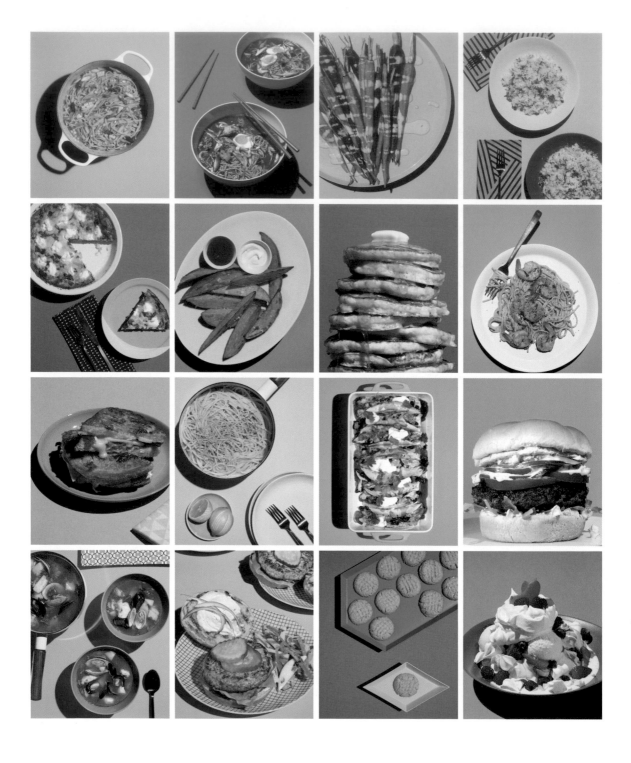

A NOTE FROM CLAUDIA FICCA

When Elettra told me about her idea to start a blog called *Impatient Foodie* that would focus on making good recipes fast, I thought it was genius! As much as I enjoy spending time in the kitchen, sometimes, after a long day's work (in the kitchen), I want to come home and make a quick, satisfying meal, dirtying the fewest number of dishes and using just a few ingredients. I often chop ingredients right over the pot to save myself from cleaning the cutting board! Elettra's impatient concept really appealed to me and writing these recipes with her has been a wonderfully delicious process. I hope this book inspires you to get in the kitchen.

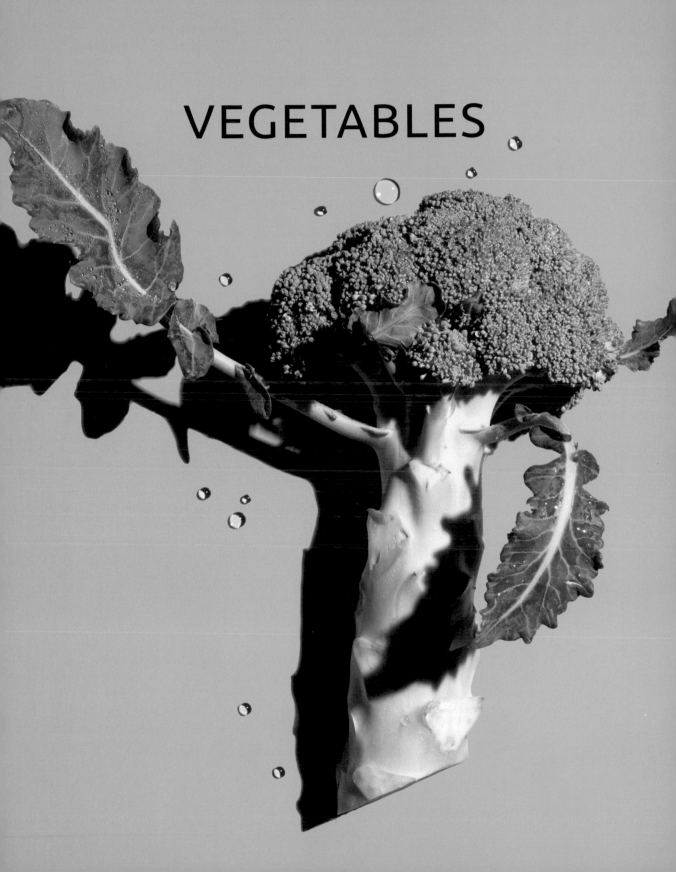

VEGETABLES

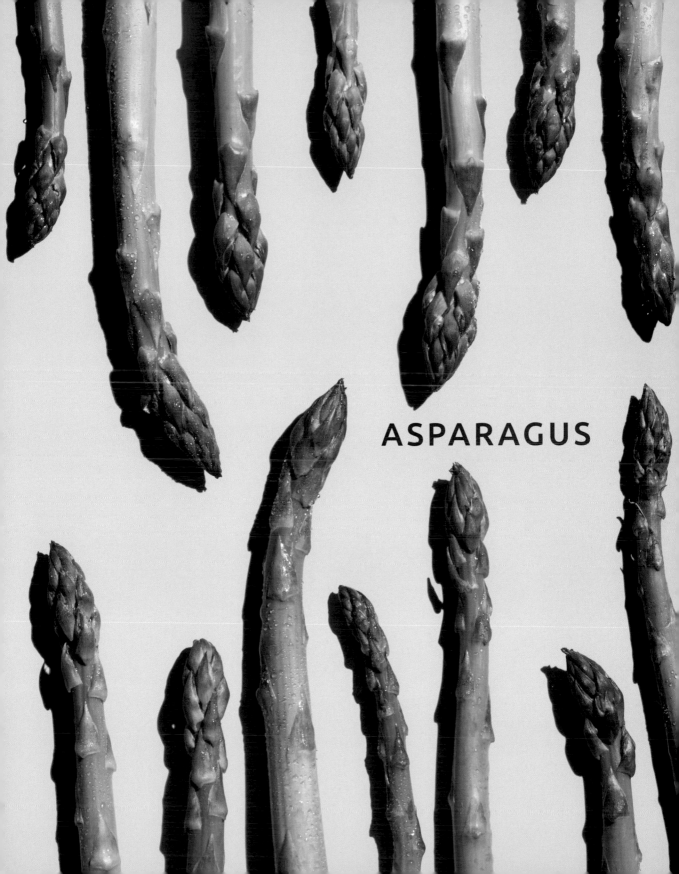

ASPARAGUS

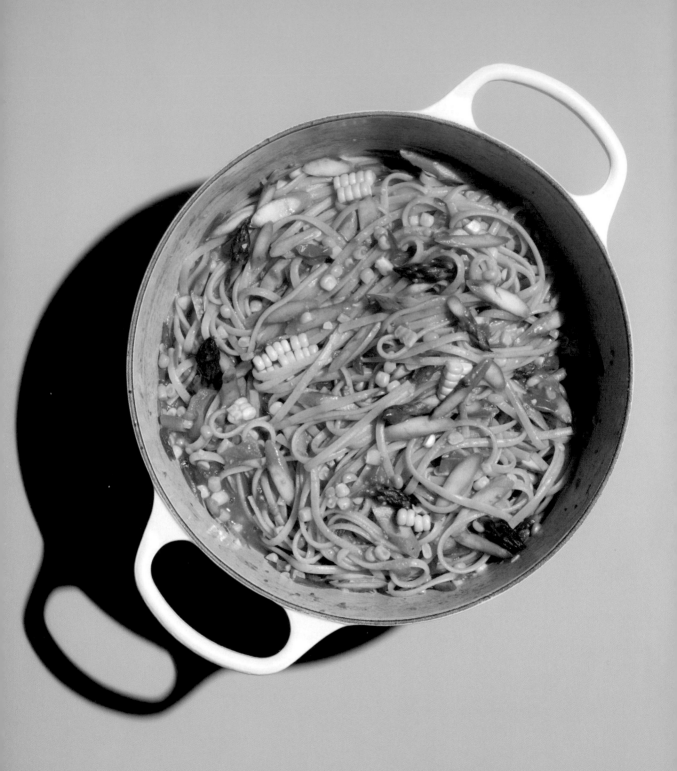

Vegan One-Pot Linguine with Asparagus and Lemon-Oregano Oil

Serves 4 to 6

This pasta is a great way to make use of the late spring, early summer bounty you can find at your farmers' market. Cooking the pasta in the sauce will give it a thicker mouth feel, which obviates the need for cheese. The lemon-oregano oil brings a nice, bright flavor to the dish.

1. Make the lemon-oregano oil: With a vegetable peeler, cut 2 large strips of zest from the lemon. In a small skillet, combine the olive oil, lemon peel, and oregano.
2. Cook over low heat until fragrant, about 15 minutes. Remove from the heat and set aside. (You will be garnishing the finished dish with this oil just before serving.)
3. Meanwhile, prepare the pasta: In a large skillet (or a Dutch oven if you have one), heat the olive oil over medium-low heat. Add the garlic and cook until fragrant, about 2 minutes. Do not allow the garlic to brown.
4. Add the tomatoes and 1 teaspoon salt, increase the heat to medium-high, and cook, stirring frequently, for 2 minutes.
5. Add 4½ cups water, cover, and bring to a boil over high heat. When it reaches a boil, add the linguine and 2 teaspoons of salt, reduce the heat to a simmer (you may have to push the linguine with the help of a wooden spoon), and cook, stirring frequently, for 15 minutes.
6. Add the asparagus and corn and stir to combine. Continue cooking for 2 to 3 minutes.
7. Plate the linguine and drizzle with 1 to 2 tablespoons of the lemon-oregano oil. Add pepper and serve.

LEMON-OREGANO OIL
1 lemon
½ cup extra virgin olive oil
1 sprig of fresh oregano

PASTA
4 tablespoons extra virgin olive oil
2 garlic cloves, minced
3 cups cherry tomatoes, halved
Kosher salt
1 pound linguine
1 bunch of asparagus, tough ends removed, spears thinly sliced on the diagonal into 1-inch lengths
Kernels from 2 ears of corn
Freshly cracked pepper

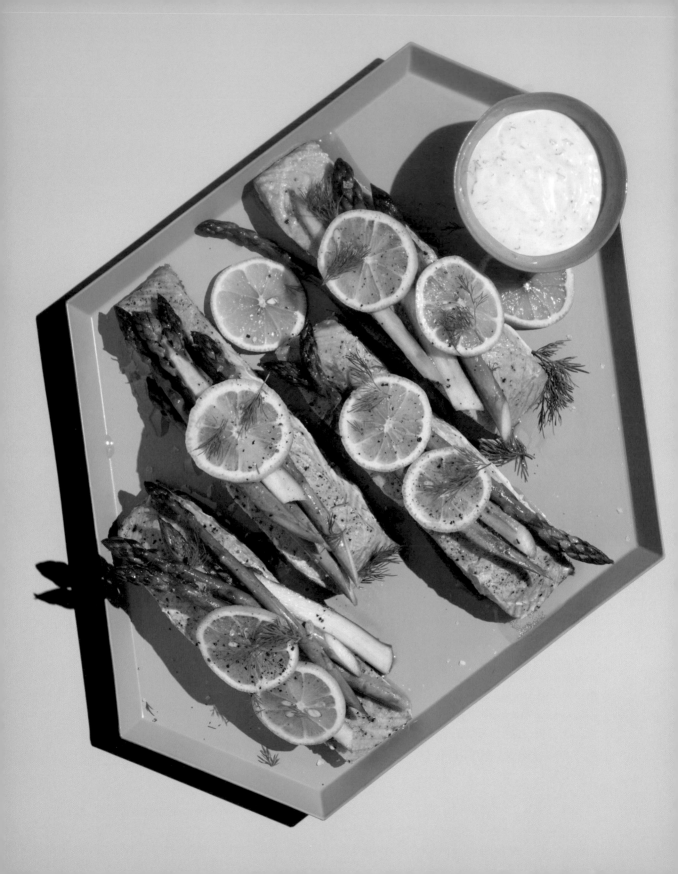

Asparagus and Salmon in Parchment with Lemon-Dill Mayo

Serves 4

I am not that great at cooking fish, but cooking it in parchment (aka en papillote) changed the game for me—it steams the fish perfectly so that it's moist and flavorful. The best part of cooking in parchment: minimal dishes.

4 (6-ounce) skinless salmon fillets

Kosher salt

16 asparagus spears, tough ends removed

3 lemons—1 juiced, 2 thinly sliced

16 small sprigs of fresh dill, plus ¼ cup chopped

2 tablespoons extra virgin olive oil

⅓ cup mayonnaise

1. Preheat the oven to 400°F.
2. Cut four 12-inch lengths of parchment paper and place on a baking sheet. Put 1 salmon fillet in the center of each piece of parchment.
3. Sprinkle each fillet with a generous pinch of salt. Lay 4 asparagus spears on top of each fillet followed by 3 lemon slices and 4 sprigs of dill. Drizzle with the olive oil.
4. To close the packets, fold the parchment over and tightly seal the edges by folding and creasing all the sides so that they are airtight but with room to allow the contents to steam properly. (Sometimes, if I am feeling especially lazy, I'll close the parchment by folding all three sides and then stapling them shut.)
5. Place the baking sheet in the oven for about 13 minutes for medium doneness.
6. Meanwhile, in a small bowl, combine the mayonnaise, lemon juice, and most of the chopped dill.
7. When time is up, remove the salmon from the oven, and split open the paper (be careful of the hot steam!). Discard the lemon and sprigs of dill.
8. Serve the salmon with a sprinkle of the remaining chopped dill, the remaining lemon slices, and a spoonful of the lemon-dill mayonnaise on the side.

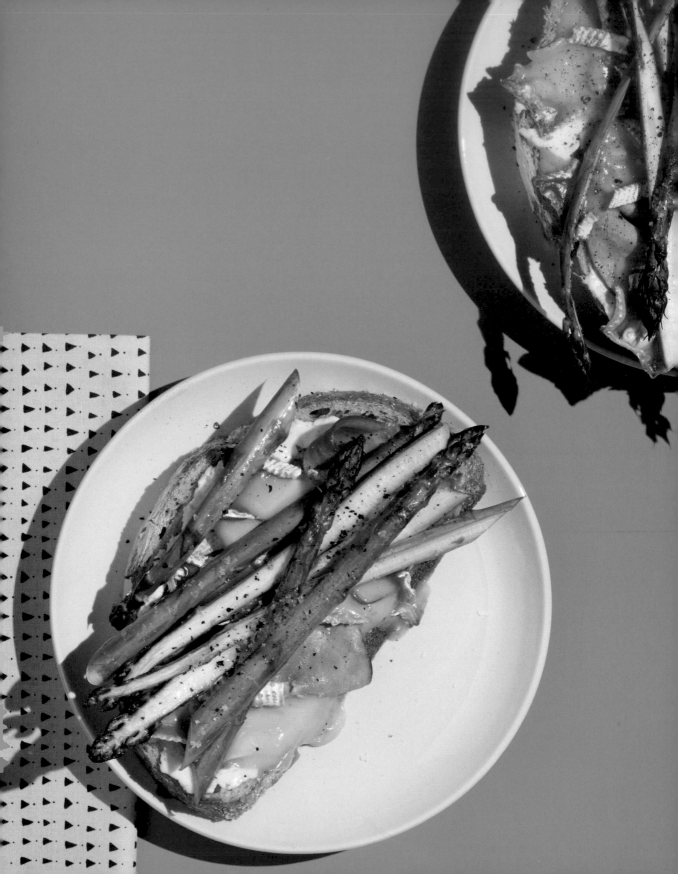

Cheesy Asparagus Tartines

Serves 4

These open-faced tartines are inspired by one of my food weaknesses—*croque monsieurs* or *croque madames*. If you are a vegetarian, you can cut out the ham.

1 bunch of asparagus, tough ends removed, spears halved lengthwise

Extra virgin olive oil

Kosher salt and freshly ground pepper

4 (1-inch-thick) slices sourdough bread (boule shaped)

1 (5.2-ounce) round Boursin cheese, quartered

8 slices cooked ham

1 (8.8-ounce) wheel Camembert cheese, cut into 12 slices

1. Preheat the oven to 375°F. Line a 15 x 10-inch baking sheet with parchment paper.
2. In a bowl, coat the asparagus with some olive oil. Add a pinch of salt and pepper and set aside.
3. To assemble the tartine, drizzle olive oil on both sides of the bread, followed by a sprinkle of salt. Spread each slice with a layer of Boursin, followed by 2 slices of ham, and topped with 3 slices of Camembert. Top the cheese with a handful of the halved asparagus.
4. Transfer the tartines to the lined baking sheet and bake for 10 minutes. Serve with pepper.

Asparagus Ribbons with Burrata and Arugula Salad

Serves 4 to 6

Extra virgin olive oil

2 bunches of asparagus (about 20 spears), tough ends removed, shaved into ribbons with a peeler

Zest of 1 lemon

1 teaspoon fresh lemon juice

4 to 6 heaping cups arugula

2 (8-ounce) containers burrata cheese, drained

¼ cup minced fresh flat leaf parsley

Balsamic glaze

Kosher salt and freshly ground pepper

Peeling asparagus ribbons is a great, impatient-friendly way to use up your bunch. I like to warm them slightly in order to soften them. The warm asparagus works nicely with the decadent, luscious burrata. Balsamic glaze is a balsamic vinegar reduction. Sweeter and more syrupy than balsamic vinegar, it's become one of my pantry staples ever since I discovered it just a few years ago—it's great on dishes like this, drizzled on salads, or even on vanilla ice cream!

1. In a medium skillet, combine 1 tablespoon of the olive oil and the asparagus ribbons and gently stir over medium-high heat until the asparagus ribbons are evenly coated in the oil. Cook the asparagus ribbons until softened, about 5 minutes. Remove from the heat and add the lemon zest and the lemon juice. Toss gently to combine.

2. Add 1 cup of arugula to each serving bowl. Dividing evenly, top the arugula with the asparagus ribbons. Break the burrata up with your hands and distribute it evenly among the bowls. Sprinkle evenly with the parsley.

3. Before serving, drizzle olive oil and balsamic glaze over the burrata and top with a pinch each of salt and pepper.

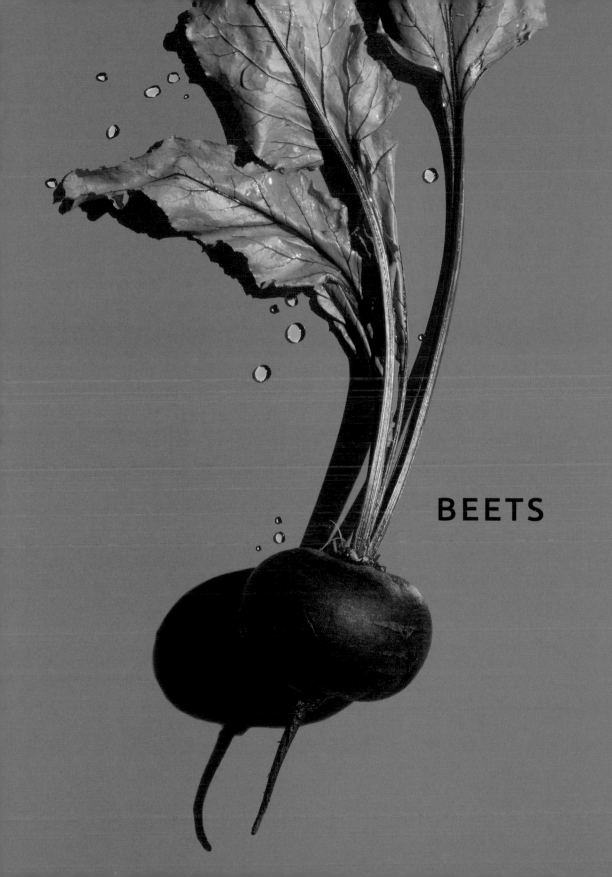

BEETS

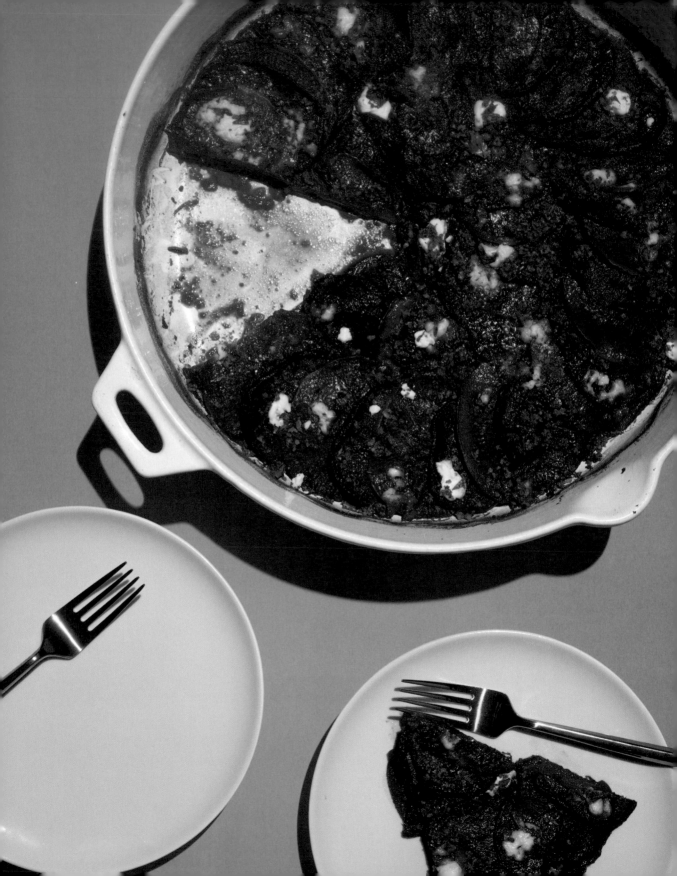

Beet Gratin with Gruyère and Goat Cheese

Serves 6 to 8

This gratin is so filling and flavorful, it can be eaten on its own or with a simple green salad as a side.

1. Preheat the oven to 400°F. Butter a large ovenproof skillet.
2. Using a mandoline, slice the beets and turnips into ⅛-inch-thick rounds.
3. Working from the outside in, make a layer of beets and turnips in the skillet, laying them in concentric circles and alternating the beets and turnips, overlapping slightly. Season with a generous pinch of salt and pepper and 1 teaspoon of the thyme. Scatter half of the Gruyère and goat cheese on top.
4. Repeat with a second layer of beets and turnips and season with a pinch of salt and pepper and the remaining 1 teaspoon of thyme. Scatter the remaining Gruyère and goat cheese on top.
5. Pour the chicken stock over everything and scatter the butter cubes evenly over the top.
6. In a bowl, mix together the bread crumbs, parsley, olive oil, and a pinch of salt and set aside.
7. Cover the skillet with foil and bake for 35 minutes. Remove the foil, scatter the bread crumb mixture on top, and bake, uncovered, until the bread crumbs brown, the juices evaporate, and a knife can easily pierce all the layers of the gratin, an additional 10 minutes. Allow to cool for 10 minutes before serving.

3 tablespoons unsalted butter, cut into cubes, plus more for greasing the skillet
5 small beets, peeled
5 small turnips, peeled
Kosher salt and freshly ground pepper
2 teaspoons fresh thyme
1½ cups grated Gruyère cheese
¼ cup crumbled goat cheese
¾ cup low-sodium chicken stock
⅓ cup unseasoned dried bread crumbs
2 tablespoons minced fresh flat leaf parsley
2 tablespoons extra virgin olive oil

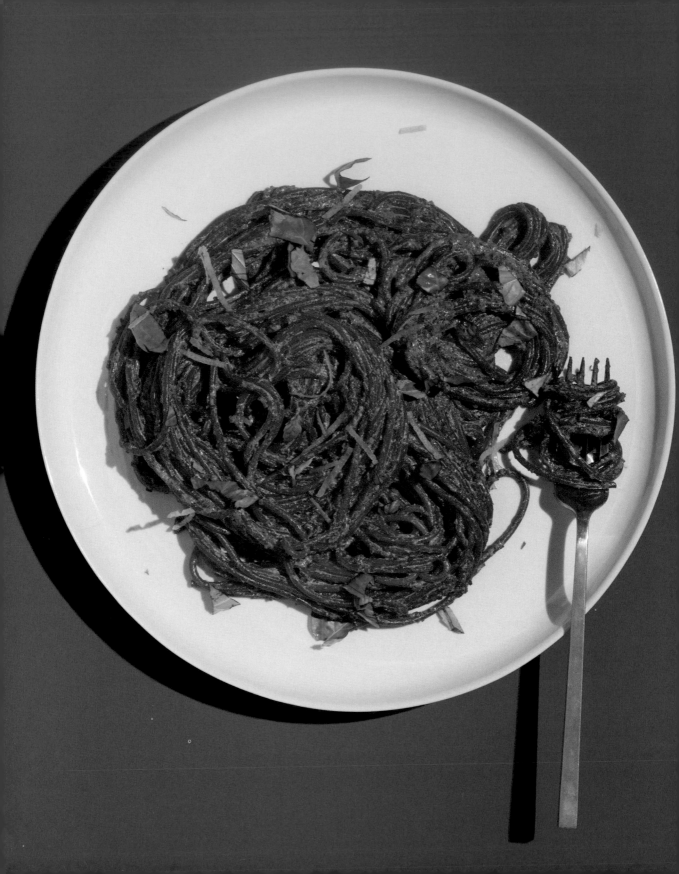

Beet and Ricotta Spaghetti

Serves 4 to 6

When cooking any pasta, salt the boiling water enough so that it takes like the sea. It'll make the spaghetti more flavorful and decrease the need for salting once the dish is served. It's also important to always cook your pasta al dente, which translates as "to the tooth." It means that well-cooked pasta should have a little "bite" to it, not be boiled to a state of mushy oblivion (unless, of course, that's how you like it, I guess?). Package directions usually indicate the cooking time for the pasta to be perfectly al dente, so no guesswork for you.

Kosher salt
2 medium beets
2 tablespoons plus ¼ cup extra
    virgin olive oil
2 cups part-skim ricotta cheese
1 pound spaghetti
½ cup chopped fresh basil
¼ cup grated Parmigiano-
    Reggiano cheese
Zest of 1 lemon (optional)

1. Bring a large pot of salted water to a boil.
2. Peel the beets and grate them on the large teardrops of a box grater. If you don't want to stain your hands, hold the beets in a piece of paper towel as you grate them.
3. In a large skillet, heat 2 tablespoons of the olive oil over medium heat. Add the grated beets and a generous pinch of salt, and cook for about 4 minutes, stirring frequently until the beets have softened. Add ½ cup of boiling water from the pot and continue to cook until the beets are very tender and the water has evaporated, about 5 minutes.
4. Transfer the cooked beets to a food processor with the remaining ¼ cup of olive oil and puree until smooth. Add the ricotta and 1 heaping teaspoon of salt. Pulse to combine. Set aside.
5. Add the spaghetti to the pot of boiling water and cook according to the package directions.
6. Reserving 1 cup of the pasta cooking water, drain the spaghetti and return it to the pot. Quickly add the beet-ricotta mixture and stir to combine. If the sauce is too thick, add some of the reserved pasta water.
7. Top with the basil, Parmigiano, and a pinch of lemon zest (if using) and serve immediately.

Beet Tahini Spread

Serves 4 to 6

2 preroasted beets, roughly
    chopped
2½ tablespoons tahini
1 tablespoon extra virgin olive oil,
    or more if needed
¼ cup canned chickpeas (garbanzo
    beans), drained and rinsed
Kosher salt and freshly ground
    pepper

This beet tahini spread is good on almost everything from toast, to roasted chicken, or even just with roasted vegetables. I have also used it as a spread on sandwiches to help reduce my compulsion to drown practically everything in mayonnaise. Preroasted beets can be purchased at some grocery stores, but if you have raw beets, you can use the impatient cooking technique we use for the Beet and Ricotta Spaghetti (page 15): Grate the beets and cook them in a skillet over medium-high heat.

In a food processor, combine the beets, tahini, olive oil, and chickpeas and puree until smooth. If more liquid is needed, slowly pour in more olive oil. Season with salt and pepper to taste and store in the fridge.

Red Beet Velvet Cake

Serves 6 to 8

If you have extra beets left over and want to do something unexpected, this is a perfect way to use them and mask their earthy
flavor in layers of sugar and deliciousness. You even use some of
the beet water to dye the icing a beautiful pink!

¾ pound (3 sticks) unsalted
butter, at room temperature,
plus more for greasing the pan
2 medium beets, peeled and cut
into 1-inch chunks
3 (8-ounce) packages cream
cheese
3 cups powdered sugar
1 tablespoon vanilla extract
1 (15.25-ounce) box chocolate
cake mix
Ingredients listed on the cake
mix package for preparing the
batter

1. Preheat the oven to 350°F. Grease two 9-inch round cake
   pans and line the bottoms with a round of parchment paper.
   Grease the parchment.
2. In a medium saucepan, combine the beets with water to
   cover. Bring to a boil, reduce the heat, and simmer until
   tender, 20 to 25 minutes.
3. Reserving ⅓ cup of the beet cooking water, drain the beets.
   (Set the tinted water aside for the frosting.) Transfer the
   beets to a food processor and process until very smooth
   (this will yield about 1 cup of beet puree). Allow to cool
   completely, about 10 minutes.
4. While the beets are cooling, make the frosting: In a large
   bowl, combine the cream cheese, butter, powdered sugar,
   vanilla, and reserved beet water and mix with a hand mixer
   until smooth. The resulting frosting should be thick and light
   pink in color. Store in the refrigerator, but remember to take
   it out 30 minutes before frosting the cake.
5. Make the chocolate cake batter according to the package
   directions and add the pureed beets as the last step, mixing
   until just combined.
6. Divide the batter between the prepared cake pans and
   bake according to the package directions (usually about
   30 minutes).
7. Let the cakes cool in the pans, about 20 minutes, then

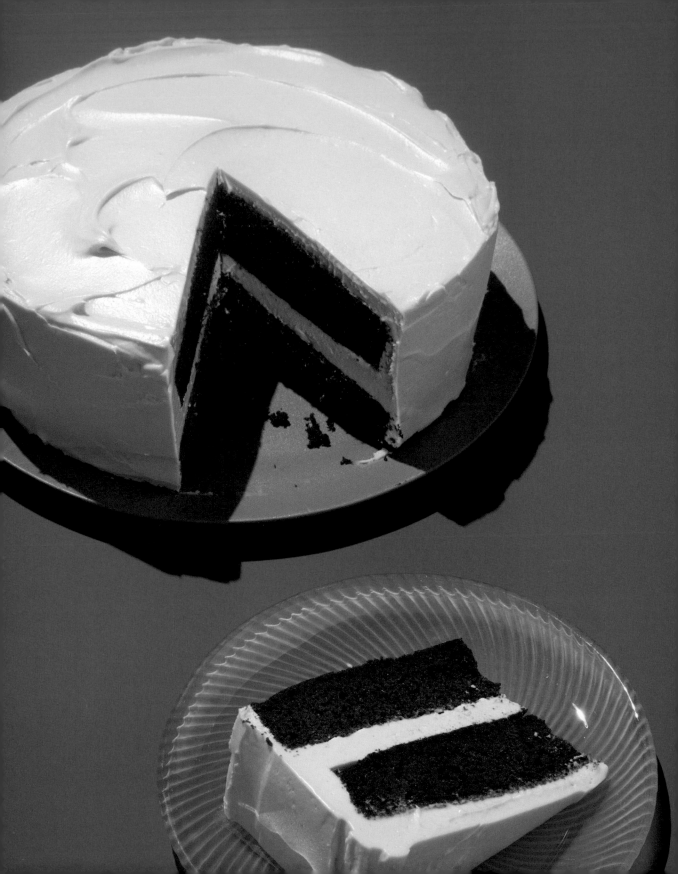

transfer the cakes to a cooling rack to cool completely before frosting. If you're impatient like me, pop them in the freezer for 15 minutes.

8. To assemble the cake, dab a small amount of frosting in the center of a flat plate (this will help keep your cake from moving around). Center the first layer of the cake on top and add 2 cups of frosting to the center of the layer. Using an offset spatula (or the back of a spoon), gently and evenly spread the icing over the bottom layer of the cake and just past the edge of the top surface.

9. Place the second layer top side down and press gently. Check to make sure it's level and centered. Add 2 cups of frosting to the center of the top layer and evenly spread it to the edges. Now frost the sides, rotating the cake as you go. Refrigerate until ready to serve.

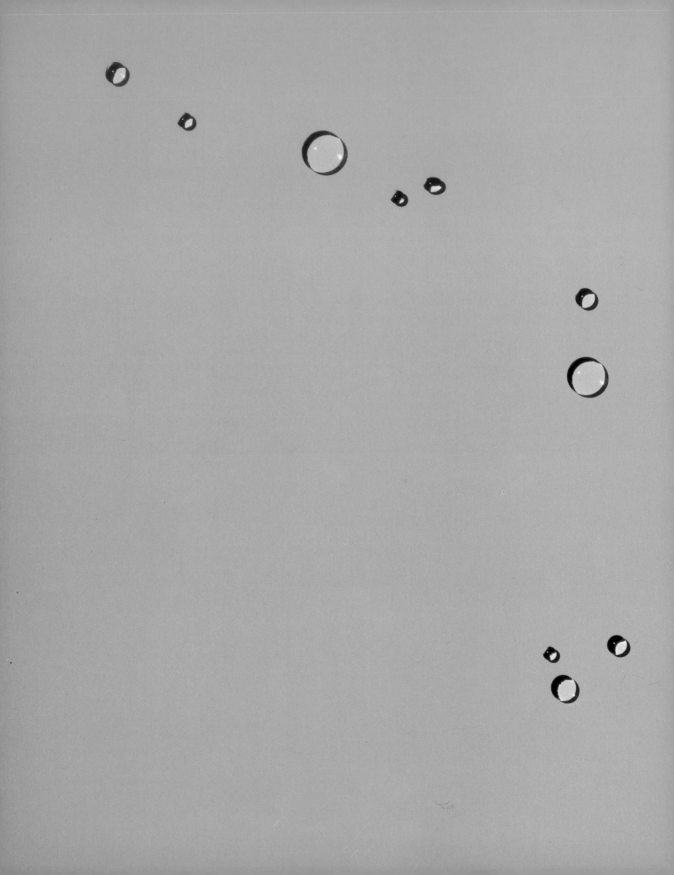

BROCCOLI

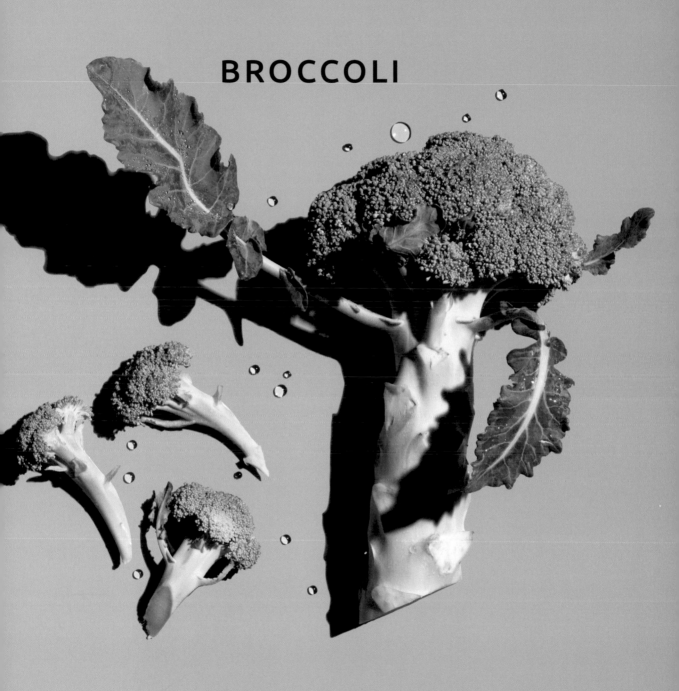

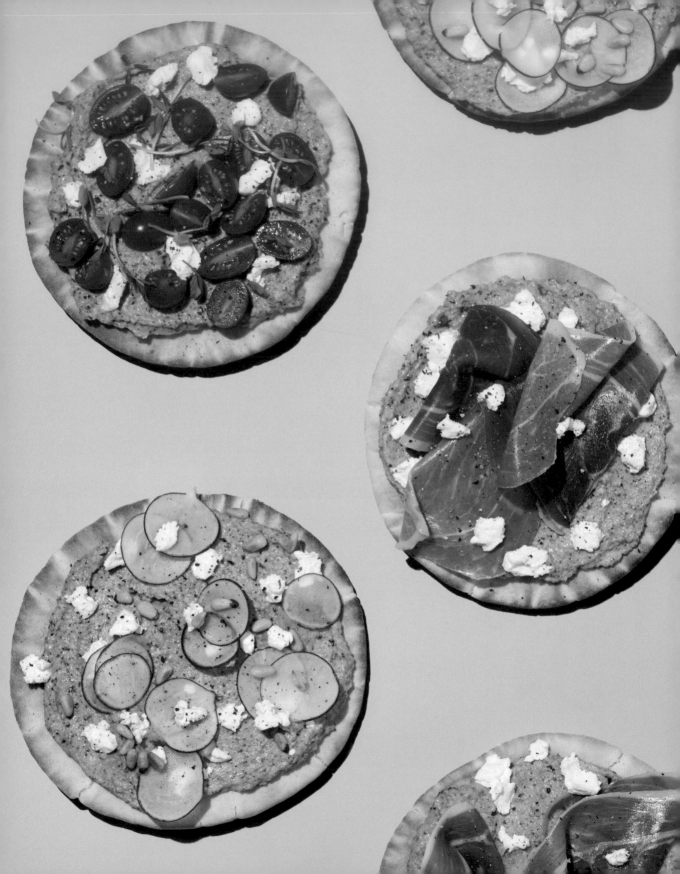

Impatient Pita Pizzas with Broccoli Pistou

Serves 6

This recipe will yield enough pistou for 12 mini pizzas plus 1¼ cups. The extra pistou can be stored in the fridge for up to a week, or frozen in an ice cube tray for use at a much later date. I use my extra pistou on pasta, on chicken, on toast with an egg on top—all scrumptious!

1. Preheat the oven to 250°F.
2. Place the pitas on a baking sheet and warm in the oven for about 5 minutes.
3. To assemble the pizzas, smear 2 tablespoons of the broccoli pistou over each warm pita bread and sprinkle with the goat cheese. Add additional toppings of your choice and enjoy.

12 (6-inch) pitas
1½ cups Broccoli Pistou (recipe follows)
2 cups crumbled goat cheese

SUGGESTED TOPPINGS (OPTIONAL)

Prosciutto
Toasted pine nuts
Sliced cherry tomatoes
Sliced radishes

Broccoli Pistou

Makes 2¾ cups

1. Bring a medium pot of water to a boil. Add the broccoli and cook until very soft, about 6 minutes. Drain the broccoli well and set aside to dry on paper towels.
2. Add the broccoli, avocado, garlic, lemon juice, basil, parsley, olive oil, salt, and Parmigiano to the food processor. Puree until smooth.

1 bunch of broccoli, cut into florets, stems peeled and chopped
1 avocado, chopped
2 garlic cloves, peeled
1 lemon, juiced
1 cup basil leaves
½ cup fresh flat leaf parsley leaves
½ cup extra virgin olive oil
½ teaspoon kosher salt
½ cup grated Parmigiano-Reggiano cheese

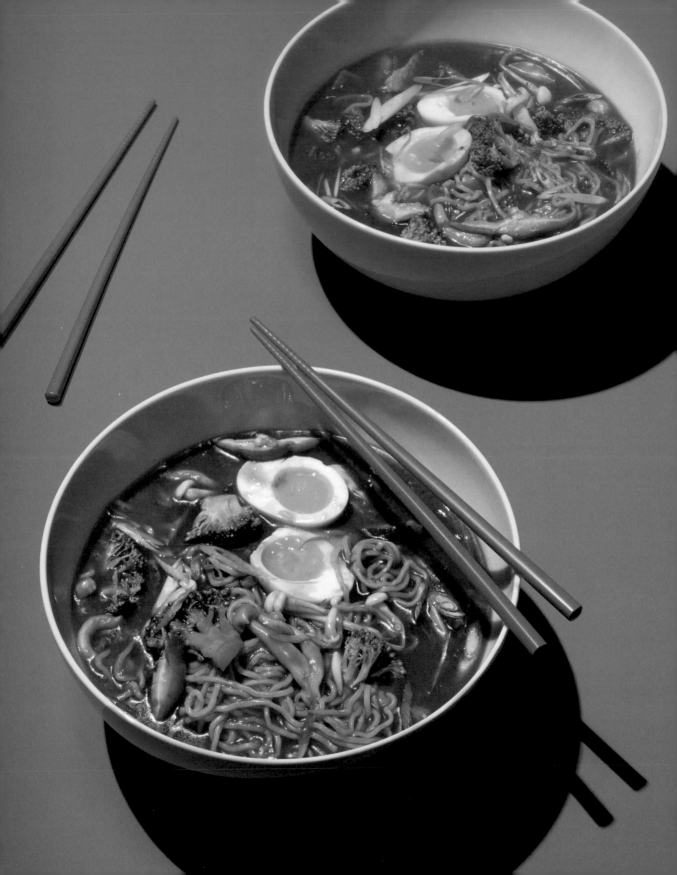

Impatient Broccoli Ramen

Serves 6

Unless you were using the just-add-water kind, making home-made ramen from scratch has been inaccessible to most home cooks, especially impatient ones. Just the tonkotsu broth alone can take days to make. And the sourcing of all the hard-to-find ingredients? Forget it! It took some experimenting, but we finally hacked a great, fast broth using beef stock as a base. The result is impatient foodie–friendly ramen anyone can make at home.

3 large eggs

2 tablespoons soy sauce

1 tablespoon toasted sesame oil

3 tablespoons white miso paste

2 garlic cloves, grated with a rasp-style zester

2 teaspoons finely grated fresh ginger

2 quarts low-sodium beef stock

Kosher salt

3 cups broccoli florets

1½ cups thinly sliced shiitake mushrooms, stems discarded

1 (3.5-ounce) package enoki or Bunapi mushrooms, stem ends trimmed

1 pound fresh ramen noodles

6 scallions, sliced, for garnish

Sriracha sauce, for serving (optional)

1. Bring a small pot of water to a boil. Place the eggs in the boiling water and cook for 6 minutes. Cool in an ice bath and peel when cool enough to handle. Set aside.

2. In a large pot, combine the soy sauce, sesame oil, miso, garlic, and ginger. Cook over low heat, stirring frequently, until fragrant, about 2 minutes.

3. Add the beef stock and 2 cups water while whisking, making sure there are no lumps. Increase the heat to high and bring to a boil.

4. Add a generous pinch of salt and taste. If the broth needs more salt, add to your liking. Add the broccoli and cook for 3 minutes, then add the mushrooms and the noodles. Stir to combine and return to a boil. Boil until the noodles are cooked, about 3 minutes.

5. Divide the noodles among bowls, top with the broth, broccoli, mushrooms, and half a soft-boiled egg per person. Sprinkle with the scallions and an artistic splatter of Sriracha (if using). Enjoy!

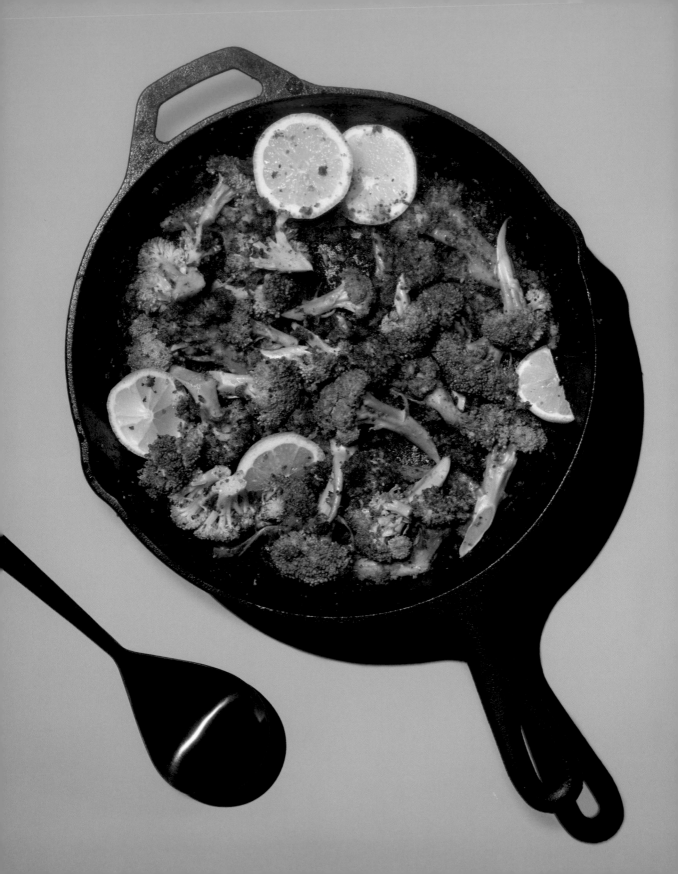

10-Minute Savory Broccoli

Serves 4 to 6

This broccoli dish is meant to be a side, but you could also toss it with some pasta and olive oil for a larger meal.

2 heads of broccoli, cut into
   florets
Kosher salt
½ cup extra virgin olive oil
2 garlic cloves, minced
2 tablespoons anchovy paste
¼ cup unseasoned dried bread
   crumbs
½ lemon, juiced

1. In a large skillet, combine the broccoli florets, ½ cup of water, and a generous pinch of salt. Bring to a boil over high heat and cover, allowing to steam for 1 to 2 minutes. Uncover and let the water evaporate from the pan.
2. Reduce the heat to medium. Add the olive oil, garlic, and anchovy paste and stir to coat the broccoli evenly. Sauté the mixture for 2 to 3 minutes.
3. Sprinkle the bread crumbs over the mixture and add 2 generous pinches of salt. Increase the heat to high and stir to coat evenly. Cook until the bread crumbs have browned, another 2 to 3 minutes.
4. Stir in the lemon juice and serve.

Raw Broccoli Salad with Sesame Dressing

Serves 4 to 6

4 to 6 cups broccoli florets, chopped

2 red, orange, or yellow bell peppers, chopped

2 avocados, roughly chopped

2 bunches of scallions, minced

1 cup raw cashews, roughly chopped

DRESSING

¼ cup toasted sesame oil

1 teaspoon rice vinegar

1 teaspoon soy sauce

1 teaspoon agave nectar

2 inches fresh ginger, peeled and grated on a rasp-style zester

½ lime, juiced

Kosher salt

Summer weather can make you feel like you are being slapped by a hot towel all day long. When it gets that hot and humid, I can't stand to eat much other than gazpacho (page 102) or a light, bright-flavored salad, like this one. This recipe is also a two-for-one! If you hold the avocado, you can sauté the rest of the salad ingredients with some sliced chicken breast and dress with the vinaigrette—an impatient stir fry!

1. In a large bowl, combine the broccoli, bell peppers, avocados, scallions, and cashews. Set aside.
2. Make the dressing: In a small bowl, whisk together the sesame oil, vinegar, soy sauce, agave, ginger, lime juice, and a pinch of salt.
3. Toss the salad with the dressing until well combined. Serve and enjoy.

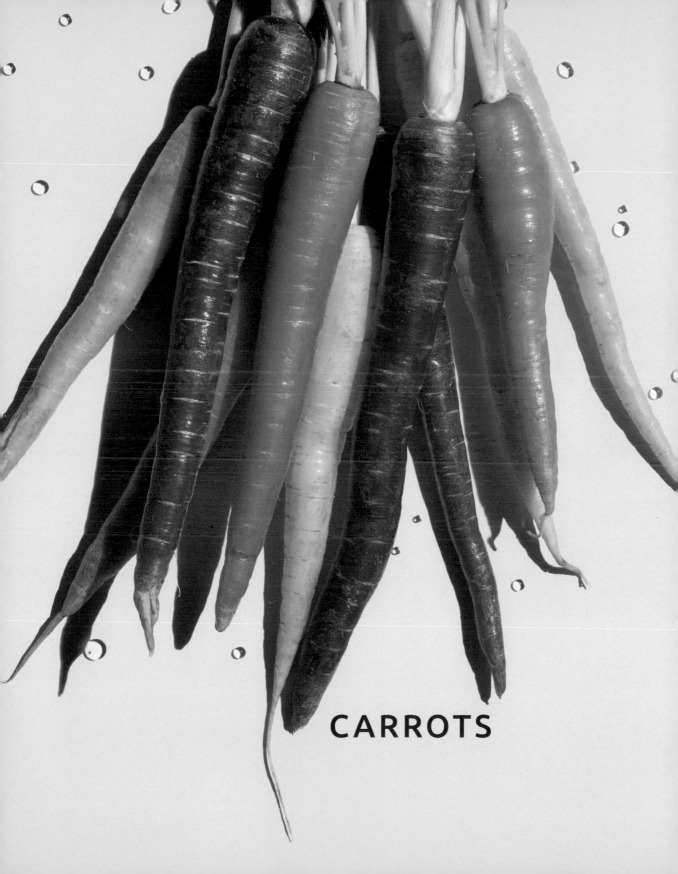

CARROTS

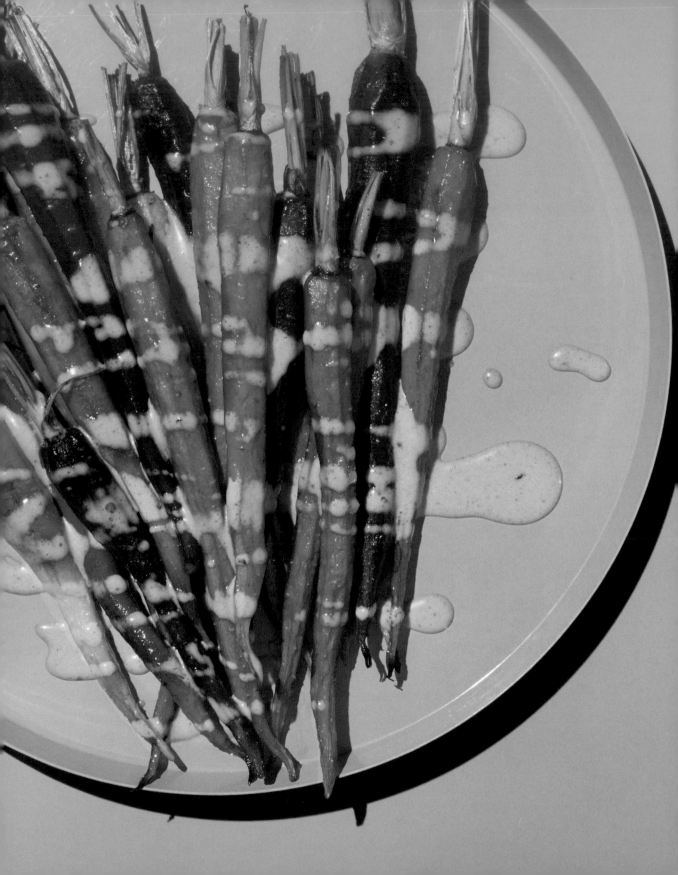

Whole Roasted Carrots with Vegan Chipotle Mayo

Serves 4

For someone who is not a trained vegan cook, making something that is completely plant based, creamy, and intensely flavorful can be a challenge. This roasted carrot dish hits all those marks. I really recommend using Hampton Creek's vegan mayonnaise—I promise you won't notice a flavor or texture difference at all.

1. To prepare the carrots: Preheat the oven to 400°F. Line a 15 x 10-inch baking sheet with parchment paper.
2. Lay the carrots on the baking sheet and pour on the olive oil and vinegar. Use your hands to make sure the carrots are evenly coated. Sprinkle evenly with salt and roast until the carrots are soft in the center when a knife is inserted, about 30 minutes.
3. Meanwhile, make the chipotle mayo: In a small bowl, stir together the mayo, adobo sauce, maple syrup, and cumin.
4. Generously drizzle the sauce over the carrots and serve.

NOTE: You can store the rest of the canned chipotle in your fridge for another use—just make sure to put it in a different container! Storing cans in the fridge is problematic because it can be toxic due to Clostridium botulinum bacterium or the metal from the can will leach into your food.

CARROTS
2 bunches of rainbow carrots, or regular carrots, peeled
2 tablespoons extra virgin olive oil
2 teaspoons balsamic vinegar
Kosher salt

CHIPOTLE MAYO
¼ cup vegan mayonnaise or regular mayonnaise (for nonvegans)
2 tablespoons adobo sauce from a can of chipotle peppers in adobo (see Note)
1 teaspoon maple syrup
¼ teaspoon ground cumin

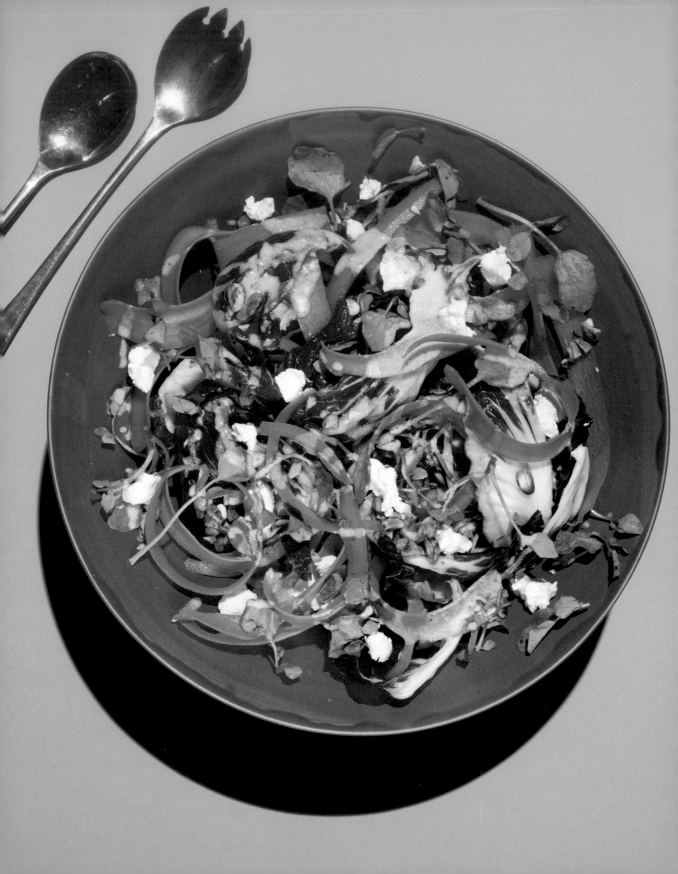

Carrot Salad with Radicchio and Feta-Pistachio Dressing

Serves 4 to 6

Many years ago, my friend showed me how to make pesto with pistachios and it was one of the best things I ever tasted. Here, we use pistachios to make a thick, creamy, nutty dressing. Paired with the sweetness of the carrots and the slight bitterness of the radicchio leaves, you'll be in heaven.

1. Make the dressing: In a food processor or blender, combine the olive oil, pistachios, tarragon, feta, lemon juice, honey, and a pinch of salt and pepper. Blend until smooth. Taste and add more salt and pepper, if desired.
2. Prepare the salad: Peel the outer leaves off of the radicchio and discard them. Fill a large bowl with cold water. Tear off the remaining radicchio leaves and place them in the cold water.
3. In a separate large bowl, shave the carrots into ribbons using a vegetable peeler.
4. Dry the radicchio and combine with the carrots. Add the watercress.
5. Pour the dressing over the carrot salad and toss until very well combined. Scatter in the feta cheese and the pistachios and serve. (If not serving immediately, store the dressing and salad separately, and dress the salad at the last minute. This will help to keep the vegetables crisp and not wilted and floppy.)

DRESSING

¾ cup extra virgin olive oil
¼ cup raw pistachios
1 tablespoon chopped fresh tarragon
2 tablespoons crumbled feta cheese
4 lemons, juiced
1 heaping teaspoon honey
Kosher salt and freshly ground pepper

SALAD

1 head of radicchio
6 large carrots, peeled
2 cups watercress
½ cup crumbled feta cheese
¼ cup raw pistachios, chopped

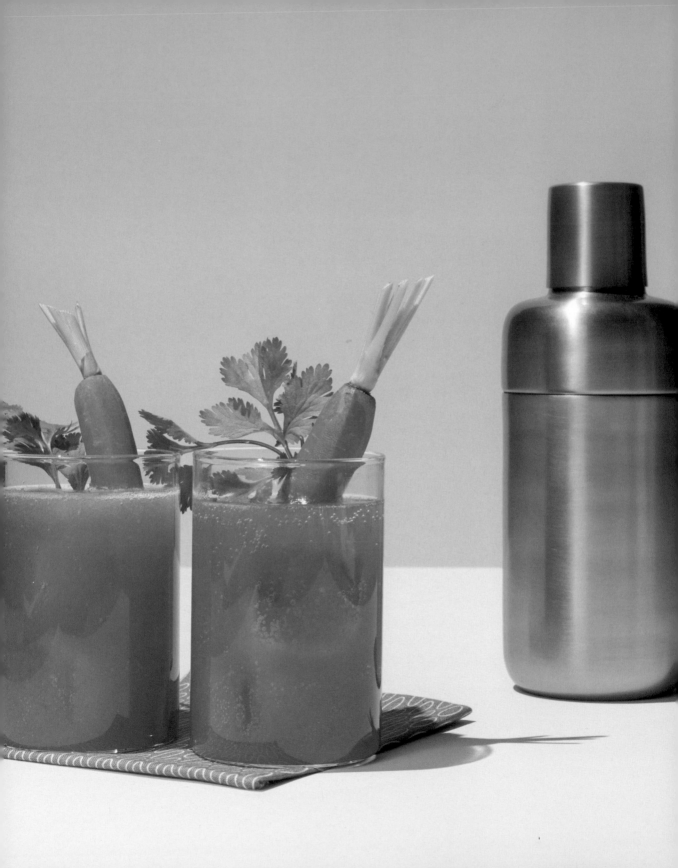

The Drunken Carrot

Makes 1 cocktail

As you can see, measurements for cocktails are in ounces, not tablespoons, teaspoons, etc.—but fear not! This is when your little measuring shot glass comes in handy! For this recipe, we used store-bought carrot-orange juice, but if you're lucky enough to have a juicer this would be even more delicious with fresh juice.

1½ ounces store-bought carrot-orange juice blend
¾ ounce fresh lime juice
½ ounce maple syrup
¾ ounce Mount Gay Barbados rum
¾ ounce Myers's dark rum
2 ounces ginger beer
1 sprig of fresh cilantro and 1 peeled baby carrot, for garnish (optional)

In a large ice-filled cup or shaker, combine the carrot-orange juice, lime juice, maple syrup, and both rums and shake. Strain into a tall ice-filled glass. Top with the ginger beer. Add a cilantro sprig and a carrot as garnish, if desired.

Carrot Mini Cupcakes with Dulce de Leche

Makes 48 mini or 24 regular cupcakes

Butter, for greasing the muffin tins

2 medium carrots, peeled

1 (15.25-ounce) box vanilla cake mix

Ingredients listed on the cake mix package for preparing the batter

1 teaspoon vanilla extract

1 teaspoon ground cinnamon

1 teaspoon ground ginger

1 (13.4-ounce) can dulce de leche

If you have two random carrots left in your fridge and you don't know what to do with them, shred them up to make these delectable two-bite mini cupcakes.

1. Preheat the oven to 350°F. Grease the cups of 2 mini or regular muffin tins or line with cupcake liners.
2. Using the small teardrops of a box grater, shred the carrots (2 medium carrots should yield about 1 cup; no worries if there is a little more or a little less).
3. In a large bowl, combine the wet ingredients called for on the cake mix package, then whisk in the vanilla, cinnamon, ginger, and shredded carrots. Add the dry cake mix and mix well to combine.
4. Divide the batter evenly among the muffin cups. Each cup should be about three-quarters full. Bake for 15 minutes for minis and 20 minutes for regular cupcakes.
5. Meanwhile, stir the dulce de leche so that it loosens up.
6. Let the cupcakes cool in the pans for 10 minutes. Remove them from the pans and top each cupcake with a dollop of dulce de leche.

CAULIFLOWER

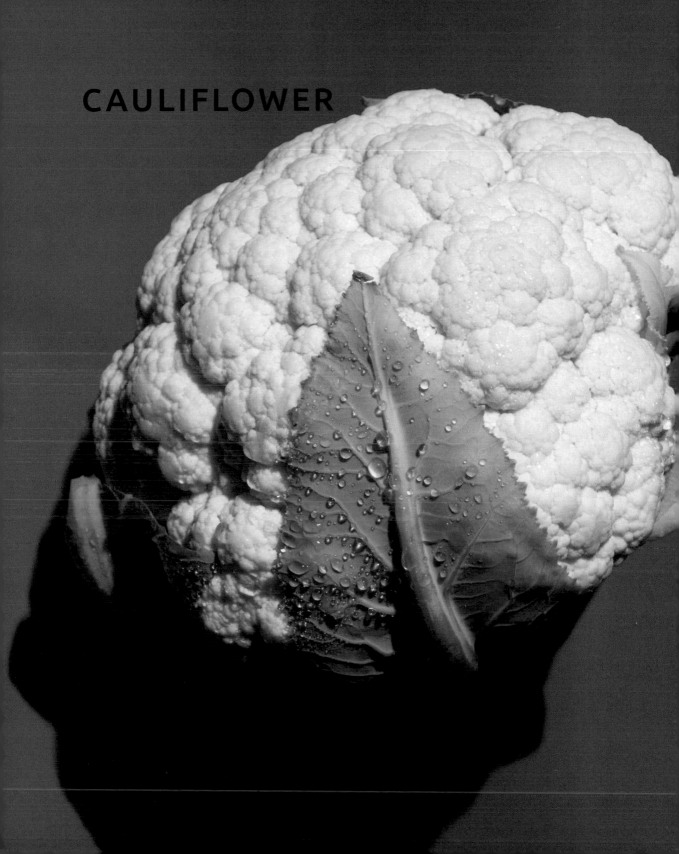

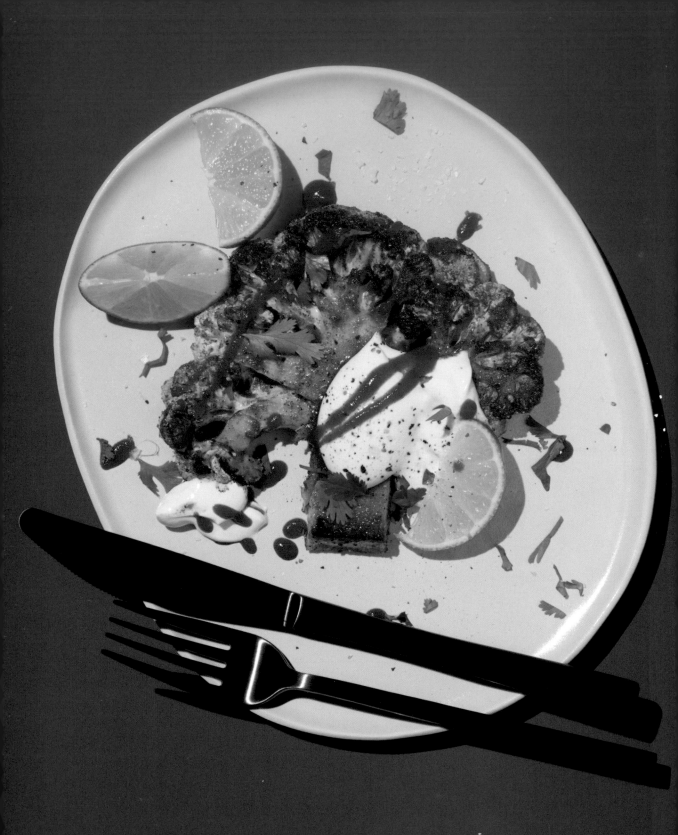

Cauliflower Steaks with Labne Cheese

Serves 4

I was late to the cauliflower steak game, but now I am a convert. Also while I am not a huge cumin fan, when everything comes together in this dish it's delicious and filling.

1. Trim the stem end of the cauliflowers to about 1 inch long, leaving the core intact. Using a large knife, cut each cauliflower from top to base, through the core, to make two 1-inch-thick steaks (4 steaks total). Use the remaining cauliflower to snack on, or in the Thai Coconut Cauliflower Soup (page 42), or add it to the crudité platter (page 99).
2. In a small bowl, whisk together 4 tablespoons of the olive oil, the cumin, coriander, turmeric, honey, and 2 generous pinches of salt.
3. Brush the cauliflower steaks with the olive oil mixture, pushing the oil into all the cauliflower's nooks and crannies.
4. In a large nonstick skillet, heat 2 tablespoons olive oil over medium-high heat. Add 2 cauliflower steaks to the skillet and cook until golden brown, 3 to 4 minutes per side. Repeat with the remaining 2 steaks.
5. Plate the cauliflower steaks and immediately sprinkle with a pinch more salt and a few turns of pepper. Then add a big dollop of labne cheese to each steak, a sprinkle of fresh cilantro, a squeeze of fresh lime juice, and a drizzle of Sriracha. Serve the remaining lime wedges on the side.

2 heads of cauliflower, leaves removed
8 tablespoons extra virgin olive oil
2 tablespoons ground cumin
1 tablespoon ground coriander
1 teaspoon ground turmeric
1 teaspoon honey
Kosher salt and freshly ground pepper

GARNISHES

Labne cheese or sour cream
½ cup chopped fresh cilantro
2 limes, quartered
Sriracha sauce

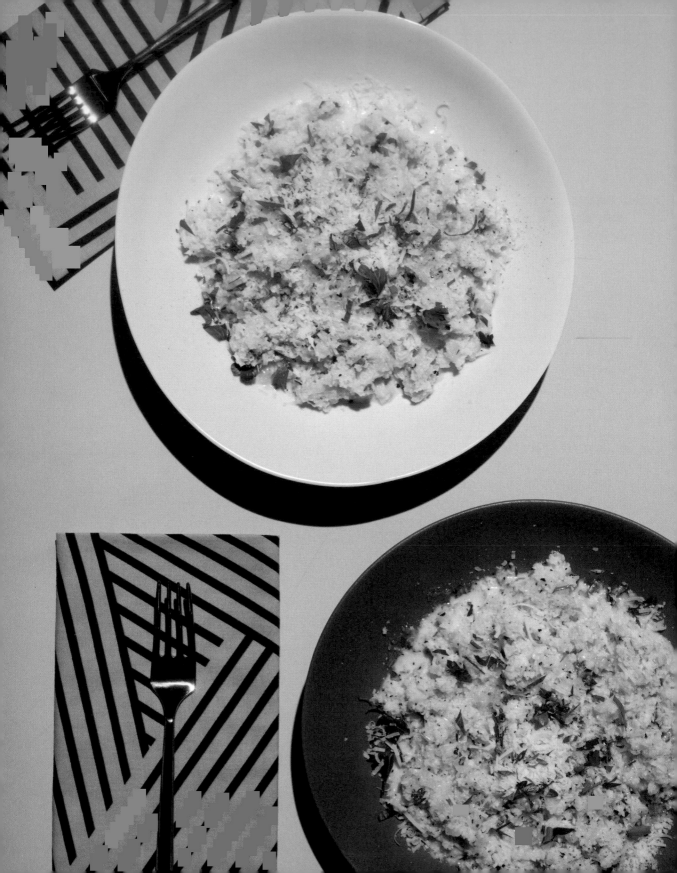

Cauliflower Risotto

Serves 4

This recipe is inspired by one of our favorite dishes at NYC's Cafe Clover. If you are gluten free, but crave some creamy, carb-y comfort, this dish is for you.

1. In a large heavy-bottomed pot, heat the olive oil over medium-high heat. Add the onion and sauté until translucent, about 3 minutes. Add a pinch of salt and the garlic and cook until fragrant, about 1 minute.
2. Add the cauliflower and sauté, stirring frequently, for 4 minutes.
3. Add the wine and cook, stirring constantly, until the wine is evaporated, about 6 minutes.
4. Add the vegetable stock, bring to a boil, then reduce the heat to low and cook the cauliflower until crisp-tender, about 5 minutes.
5. Transfer 2 cups of the cauliflower to a blender, add ¼ cup of water, and puree until smooth. Transfer the pureed cauliflower back to the pot and stir in the cream, Parmigiano, truffle oil, and butter until well combined.
6. Serve garnished with parsley and a drizzle of olive oil. Sprinkle with some more Parmigiano, if desired.

6 tablespoons extra virgin olive oil, plus more for drizzling
1 medium yellow onion, minced
Kosher salt
4 garlic cloves, minced
2 heads of cauliflower, grated on the large teardrops of a box grater (8 to 10 cups)
2 cups white wine
1 cup low-sodium vegetable stock
6 tablespoons heavy cream
½ cup grated Parmigiano Reggiano cheese
½ teaspoon truffle oil
4 tablespoons (½ stick) unsalted butter
½ cup fresh flat leaf parsley, minced

Thai Coconut Cauliflower Soup

Serves 2 to 4

2 tablespoons extra virgin olive oil

2 shallots, sliced

1 medium head of cauliflower, broken into florets

2 cups low-sodium vegetable stock or water

1 (13.5-ounce) can unsweetened coconut milk

3 tablespoons soy sauce

1 teaspoon kosher salt

2 tablespoons red curry paste

2 limes, quartered

2 tablespoons chopped fresh cilantro

1 scallion, sliced

This quick and easy soup takes twenty minutes and its surprising flavor combination will make cauliflower one of your favorite veggies.

1. In a large pot, combine the olive oil and shallots and sauté over medium-low heat until the shallots are soft and translucent, about 3 minutes.

2. Add the cauliflower, vegetable stock, coconut milk, soy sauce, salt, and curry paste and stir to combine. Bring to a boil, then reduce the heat to a simmer, cover, and cook until the cauliflower is very soft, about 15 minutes.

3. Remove from the heat and puree the soup with an immersion blender or regular blender. Taste the soup and add more soy sauce, if desired.

4. Serve the soup with a lime wedge, and garnish with cilantro and scallion.

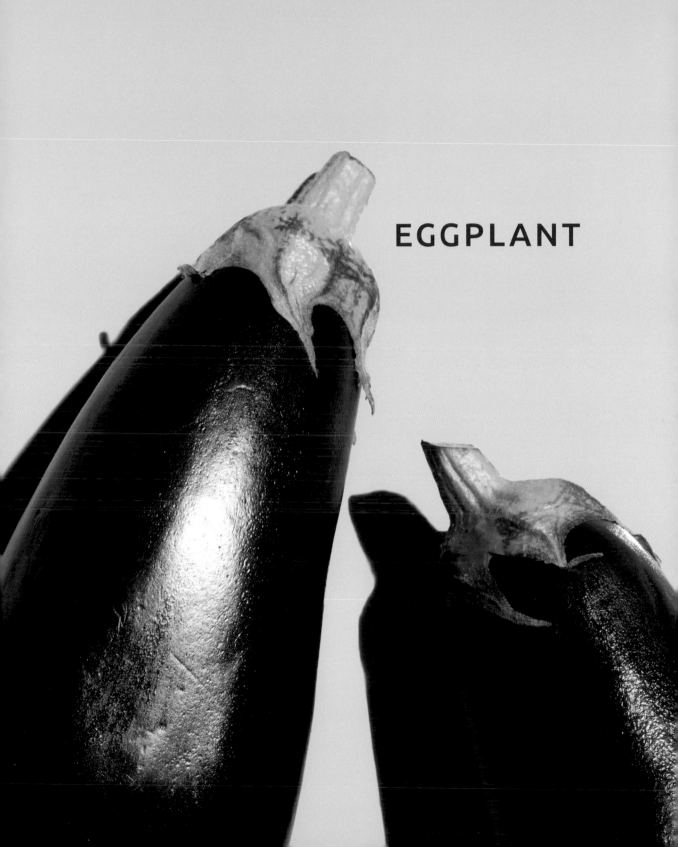

EGGPLANT

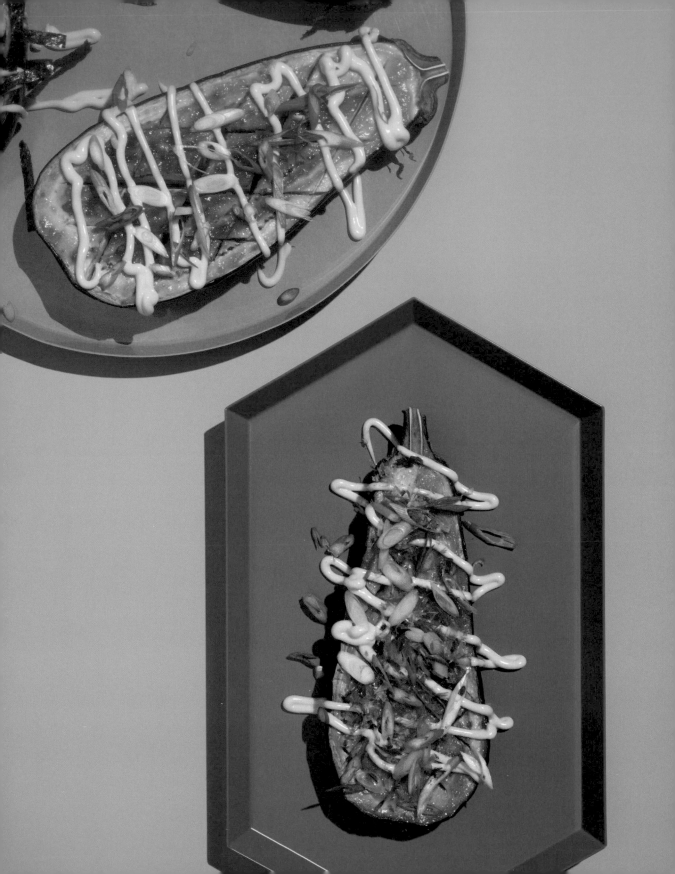

Miso-Braised Eggplant

Serves 2 to 4

Kewpie mayonnaise is a Japanese brand that comes in a squeez-able bottle with a small dispenser head. If you don't want to go out and find Kewpie, that is totally fine—any regular mayo will do. You can create the drizzle effect by piping the mayo of your choice out of a zip-seal plastic bag with a tiny hole cut in the cor-ner.

2 medium eggplants, unpeeled
Kosher salt
2 teaspoons toasted sesame oil
2 teaspoons ume plum vinegar
2 teaspoons honey
2 tablespoons white miso paste
Mayonnaise, preferably Kewpie

TOPPINGS (OPTIONAL)
2 scallions, sliced diagonally
Bonito flakes
1 (0.35-ounce) package roasted sesame seaweed snack, cut into thin strips

1. Preheat the oven to 375°F. Line a 15 x 10-inch baking sheet with parchment paper.
2. Halve the eggplants lengthwise. Score the eggplant flesh with diagonal incisions, being careful not to pierce the skin.
3. Place the eggplants on the lined baking sheet cut side up. Sprinkle each eggplant with salt.
4. In a small bowl, combine the sesame oil, vinegar, honey, and miso. Whisk together to make a paste. Spoon equal amounts of the miso mixture over each eggplant half and spread to coat evenly.
5. Bake until tender, 40 to 45 minutes.
6. Let the eggplants cool for 5 minutes. Drizzle the mayo over the eggplants. If desired, top with a sprinkle of scallions, bonito flakes, and/or seaweed strips.

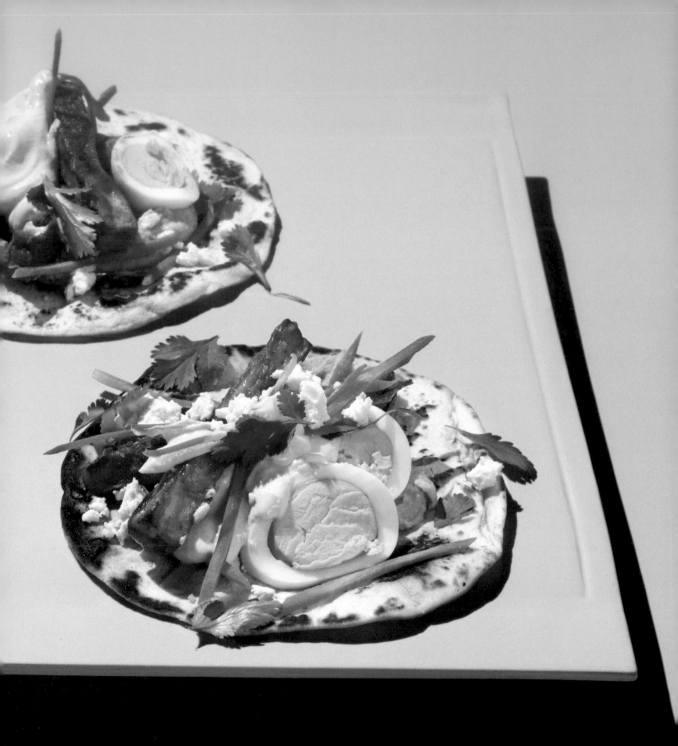

Eggplant Tacos

Serves 4 to 6

Multiple dishes that need washing is a price I am willing to pay for homemade tacos. This recipe replaces meat with thick-cut baked eggplant fries. The result is a filling, hearty, vegetarian-friendly taco everyone can enjoy.

1. Preheat the oven to 400°F. Line a 15 x 10-inch baking sheet with parchment paper.
2. Make the eggplant fries: Slice the eggplant into fry shapes, about 3½ inches long and ½ inch thick.
3. In a medium bowl, stir together the flour, paprika, cayenne, and salt.
4. In a separate bowl, whisk together 1 egg and 1 tablespoon of the olive oil.
5. One at a time, dip the eggplant fries into the egg mixture first, then dredge in the flour mixture and place on the lined baking sheet. Coat the eggplant fries with a light coating of olive oil spray.
6. Bake until the fries are crispy and golden brown, about 20 minutes, turning once midway through.
7. Meanwhile, make the sauce: In a small bowl, whisk together the yogurt, Sriracha, and lemon juice. Set aside.
8. Prepare the taco fillings: Bring a medium pot of water to a boil. Gently drop in the eggs. Set a timer for 10 minutes. Immediately remove the eggs from the hot water and run them under cold water. Once cooled, gently roll the eggs on a hard surface to break their shells and peel them. Slice the eggs and set aside.
9. When the eggplant fries are done, remove them from the oven and allow them to cool slightly. Turn the oven off, but

BAKED EGGPLANT FRIES

1 medium eggplant, peeled
1½ cups all-purpose flour
1 teaspoon paprika
¼ teaspoon cayenne pepper
½ tablespoon kosher salt
1 large egg
1 tablespoon extra virgin olive oil
Olive oil spray

SPICY YOGURT SAUCE

1 cup full-fat Greek yogurt
½ tablespoon Sriracha sauce
1 lemon, juiced

TACO FILLINGS

4 large eggs
12 (6-inch) flour tortillas (fajita size)
¾ cup store-bought plain hummus
2 medium carrots, grated (about 1 cup)
6 tablespoons crumbled feta cheese
6 tablespoons chopped fresh cilantro

place the tortillas directly on an oven rack in the warm oven for 2 minutes—set a timer!

10. To assemble the tacos, smear 1 tablespoon of hummus in the center of each tortilla, followed by 2 to 3 eggplant fries, grated carrots, several slices of egg, and ½ tablespoon of feta. Top with the cilantro. As a final touch, drizzle the spicy yogurt sauce over the tacos. Serve immediately.

Impatient Eggplant Fusilli

Serves 4 to 6

Apart from draining hot water into a colander, this fusilli dish all gets cooked and mixed together in just one pot. It's a delicious, unexpected, and impatient way to make use of and cook up eggplants, which are usually a little on the "high maintenance" side.

2 tablespoons extra virgin olive oil, plus more for drizzling

4 garlic cloves, thinly sliced

1 pound fusilli

1 medium eggplant, unpeeled, cut into ½-inch cubes

Kosher salt

1 cup grated pecorino cheese, some reserved for garnish

1 lemon, zested and juiced

3 tablespoons heavy cream

1 cup fresh flat leaf parsley, chopped

Freshly ground pepper

1. In a large pot, heat the olive oil over medium-low heat, add the garlic, and sauté until fragrant, 1 to 2 minutes.
2. Add the fusilli and eggplant cubes along with 2 tablespoons kosher salt and 8 cups water. Bring to a boil over high heat. Cover, reduce the heat to a simmer, and cook until fusilli is al dente, 10 to 12 minutes.
3. Drain the fusilli and eggplant and return to the same hot pot. Add all but a small amount of the pecorino, the lemon zest, lemon juice, cream, and parsley. Mix together very well before tasting. Add salt and pepper to taste.
4. Serve with a sprinkle of the remaining pecorino on top plus a drizzle of olive oil, if desired.

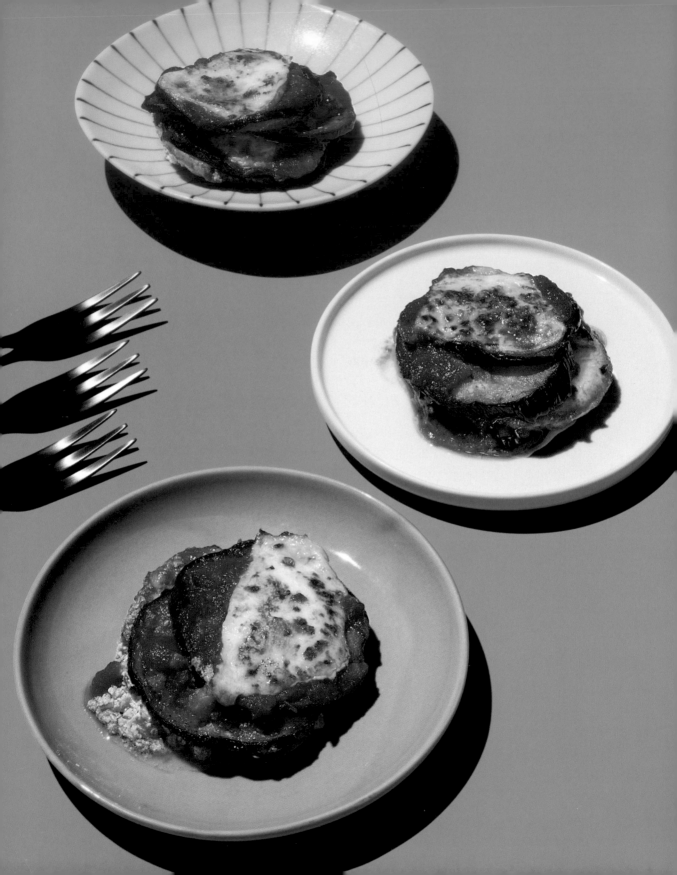

Muffin-Tin Eggplant Parmigiana

Makes 12 eggplant Parmigiana "muffins"

This is Claudia's eggplant Parmigiana hack: By cutting things up small and baking them in a muffin tin, the prep time goes down considerably, as does your cooking time.

1. Preheat the oven to 375°F. Evenly coat a 15 x 10-inch baking sheet with the 2 tablespoons of olive oil.
2. Place the eggplant slices in one layer on the oiled baking sheet and flip to coat both sides. Season all the eggplant slices with an even sprinkle of salt.
3. Bake until the eggplant is soft and malleable, about 15 minutes.
4. Meanwhile, grease 12 cups of a muffin tin with olive oil.
5. Remove the eggplant from the oven and reduce the oven temperature to 350°F.
6. In a medium bowl, stir together the ricotta, basil, pepper, and ½ teaspoon salt.
7. Assemble the ingredients in the following order in the muffin cups:

   - 1 teaspoon marinara sauce
   - 2 slices baked eggplant
   - 1 heaping tablespoon ricotta mixture
   - 1 slice mozzarella

   Repeat the layering.
8. Bake until the mozzarella is browned and the sauce is bubbling, about 30 minutes. Allow to cool slightly before removing from the muffin tin.

2 tablespoons extra virgin olive oil, plus more for greasing the muffin tins

3 small eggplants, unpeeled, thinly sliced in rounds (you should have 16 slices per eggplant for 4 slices of eggplant per muffin cup)

Kosher salt

1½ cups whole-milk ricotta cheese

¼ cup chopped fresh basil

¼ teaspoon freshly ground pepper

½ cup high-quality marinara sauce (we like Mario Batali's; store leftover sauce for another use)

½ pound mozzarella cheese, quartered and sliced (you need 24 slices)

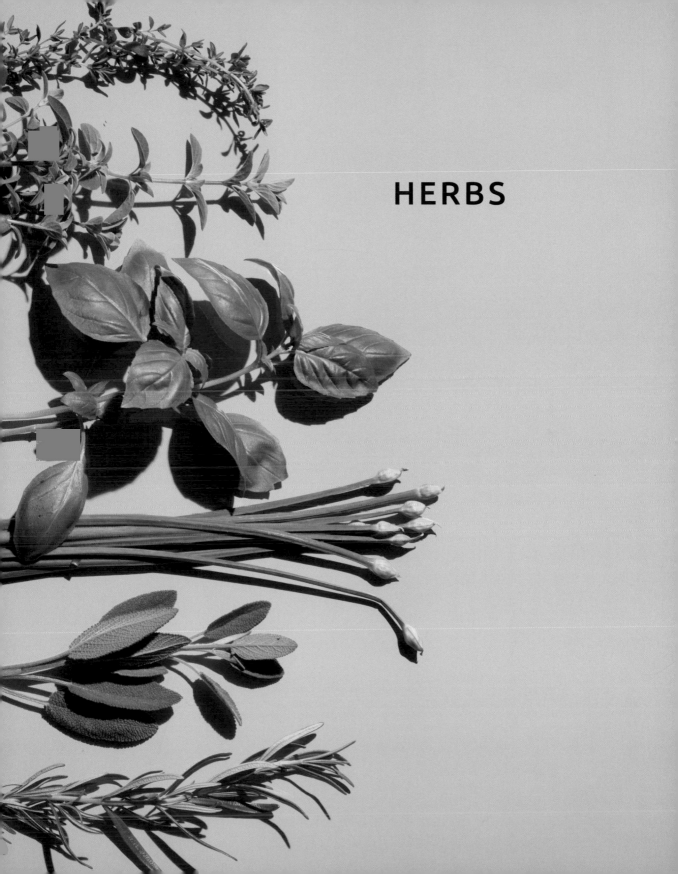

HERBS

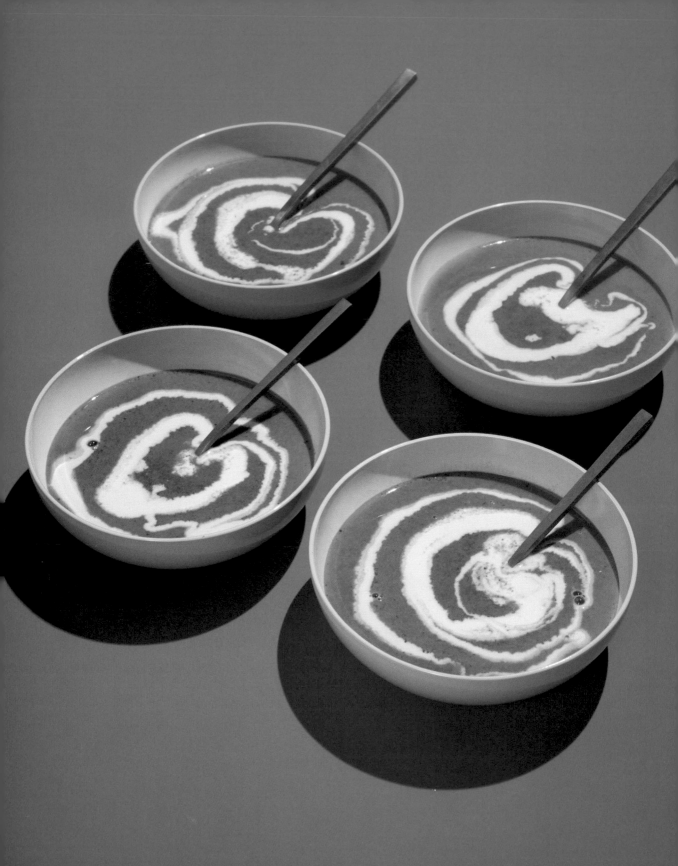

Eat Your Veggies Soup

Serves 2 to 4

This soup is a great way to make use of the greens and leftover herbs (like basil, sage, dill) that are languishing in your fridge. It can also be made without herbs, if you don't have any lying around.

2 tablespoons extra virgin olive oil
2 garlic cloves, minced
1 small yellow onion, diced
2 cups low-sodium vegetable stock
1 large handful of spinach
2 large handfuls of arugula
Leftover herbs (optional)
½ lemon, juiced
Kosher salt and freshly ground
    pepper
Crème fraîche, for garnish
    (optional)

1. In a large pot, heat the olive oil over medium-high heat. Add the garlic and onion and sauté until the onions are softened and translucent, 3 to 4 minutes.
2. Pour in the vegetable stock and bring to a boil. Add in the spinach, arugula, and up to 1 cup of mixed leftover herbs like basil, parsley, oregano, cilantro, or marjoram, if using. (I would avoid rosemary as it will overpower the soup.) Cook until the arugula and spinach are just wilted, about 2 minutes. Add the lemon juice and a generous pinch of salt and pepper. Stir to combine.
3. Puree the soup with an immersion blender or regular blender. Transfer the soup to serving bowls and garnish with a little crème fraîche, if desired.

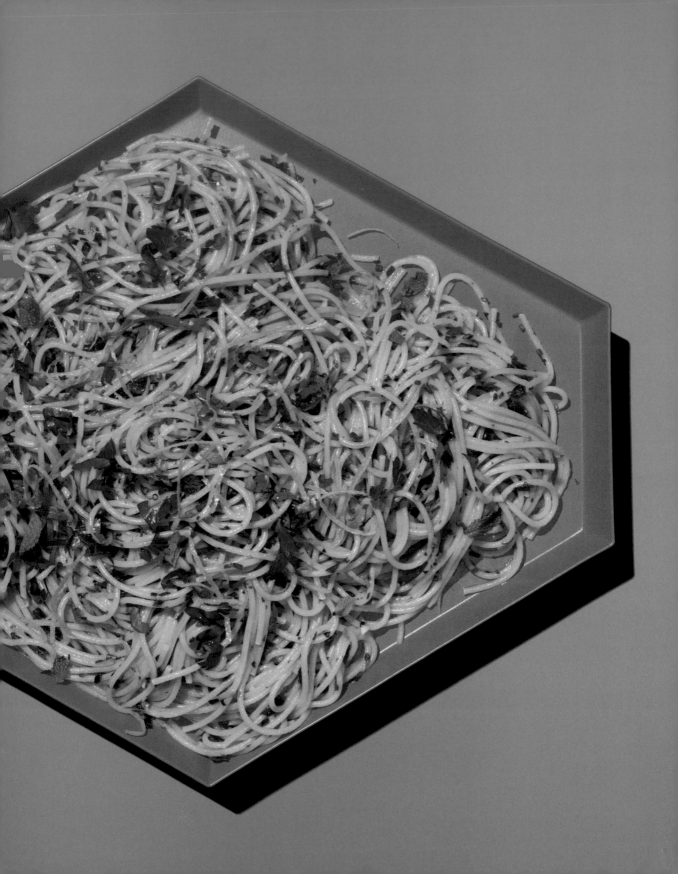

Rossellini Spaghetti

Serves 4 to 6

This recipe was invented by my grandfather, Roberto Rossellini, and passed down to my mom and her siblings. My mom makes this in the summer to use up any leftover or excess herbs. You can use any herbs you have on hand and adjust the amount according to your taste; for example, if you don't like oregano, you can skip it all together. The light, fragrant flavor of this spaghetti dish makes this a family favorite for hot weather. My grandfather also invented this recipe while keeping his hatred of doing the dishes in mind—genius (and clearly impatience runs in my blood going way back!).

Kosher salt

1 pound spaghetti

1 cup finely chopped fresh basil

1 cup finely chopped fresh flat leaf parsley

1 cup finely chopped fresh chives

¼ cup finely chopped fresh sage

½ cup finely chopped fresh mint

¼ cup finely chopped fresh oregano

Zest of 1 lemon

1 cup extra virgin olive oil

1 garlic clove, minced (optional)

1 cup grated Parmigiano-Reggiano cheese

Freshly ground pepper

1. Bring a large pot of salted water to a boil. Add the spaghetti and cook according to the package directions.
2. Meanwhile, place all the chopped herbs in a serving bowl with the lemon zest, olive oil, garlic (if using), half of the Parmigiano, and a generous pinch of salt and pepper.
3. Drain the spaghetti and transfer immediately to the serving bowl with the herbs. Toss together until the spaghetti is evenly coated with olive oil and herbs. Top with the remaining Parmigiano before serving and enjoy immediately.

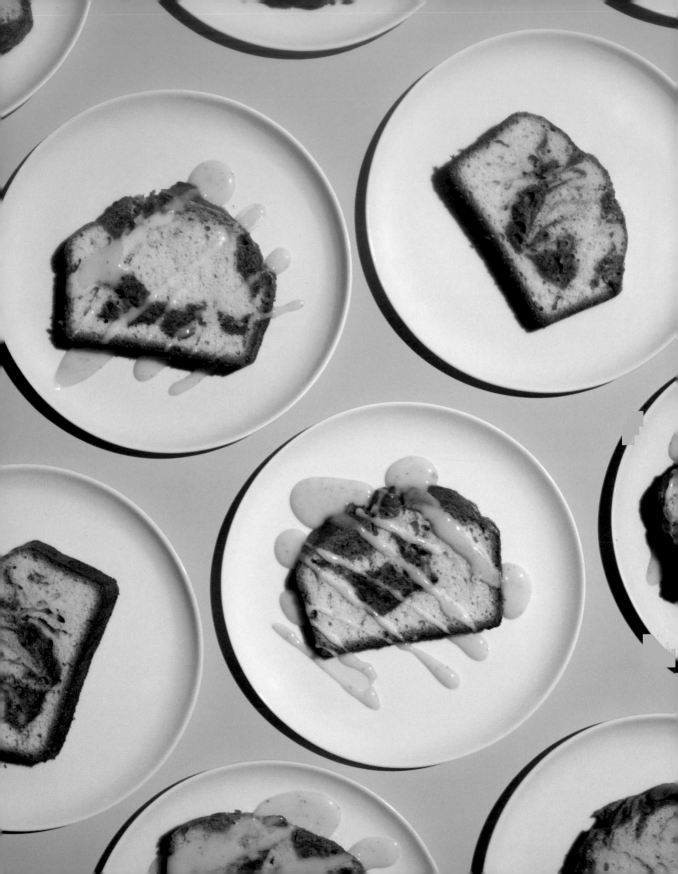

Raspberry-Almond Marble Cake with Basil Glaze

Serves 6 to 8

Basil is usually used as a garnish or in a sauce, but we found that it was the perfect flavor accent for this pound cake made with raspberry jam and almond butter.

1. Preheat the oven to 350°F. Grease a 9 x 5 x 3-inch loaf pan and set a piece of parchment paper inside so that the parchment hangs over the long sides of the loaf pan. Grease the parchment lightly.
2. In a large bowl, make the pound cake batter according to the package directions.
3. In a separate bowl, mix together the raspberry jam and almond butter. Fold in 1 cup of the pound cake batter.
4. Spread 2 cups of the pound cake batter into the loaf pan and dollop with ½ cup of the raspberry-almond batter. Drag and swirl the tip of a knife through the batter to create a marble effect. Add the remaining pound cake batter and spread evenly, then top with the rest of the raspberry-almond batter and repeat the marble effect.
5. Bake according to the package directions (usually 50 to 60 minutes) until the top is golden brown and a toothpick comes out clean. Allow the pound cake to cool in the loaf pan for 20 minutes. Remove the pound cake from the loaf pan by pulling up the parchment paper and transfer it to a cooling rack to cool completely.
6. Meanwhile, make the glaze: In a small bowl, whisk together the milk, basil, powdered sugar, lemon zest, and a pinch of salt.
7. Strain the glaze through a sieve to remove the basil leaves. Drizzle the glaze over the pound cake. Enjoy!

Butter or coconut oil, for greasing the pan
1 (16-ounce) box plain pound cake mix
Ingredients listed on the cake mix package for preparing the batter
½ cup raspberry jam
⅓ cup almond butter

GLAZE

3 tablespoons whole milk
3 tablespoons minced fresh basil
1 cup powdered sugar
Zest of 1 lemon
Kosher salt

I Can't Believe It's Vegan Pesto

Makes about 1 cup

¼ cup raw cashews
¼ cup raw pistachios
½ cup extra virgin olive oil, or
    more if needed
1½ to 2 heaping cups fresh basil
    leaves
1 garlic clove, peeled
1 lemon, juiced
Kosher salt

This recipe can easily be doubled or tripled. I am mildly addicted to this so I make a lot and store it in my fridge and freezer. I find this pesto goes with pretty much everything. Sometimes I just eat it by the spoonful!

1. In a food processor, puree the cashews, pistachios, olive oil, basil, garlic, half of the lemon juice, and a generous pinch of salt until completely smooth. If the mixture looks too dry, add 2 to 3 more tablespoons of olive oil.
2. Taste the pesto and add more of the lemon juice and salt if needed, adding a little at a time. It can be used immediately, stored in the fridge for up to 1 week, or frozen.

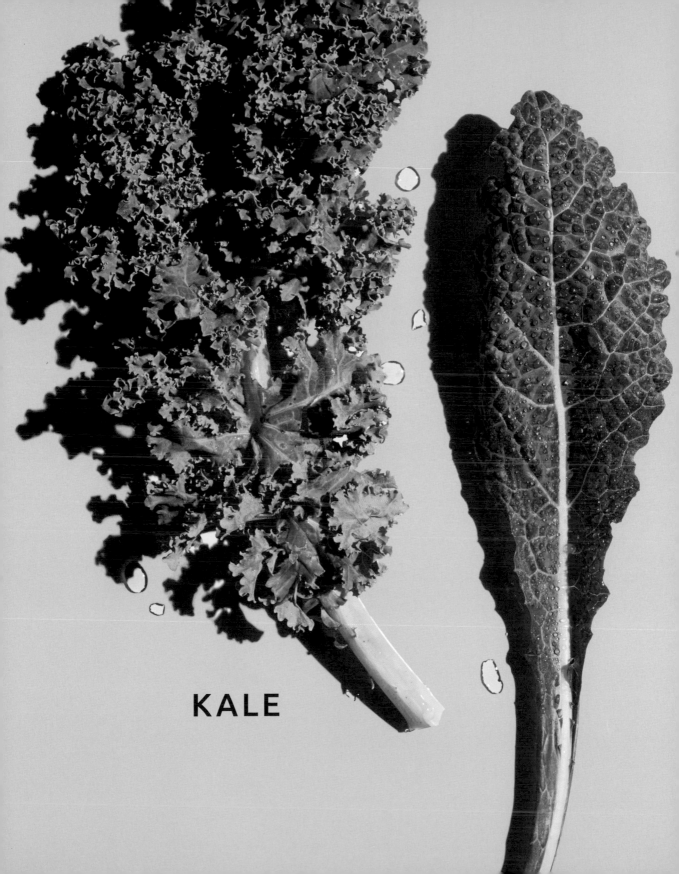

KALE

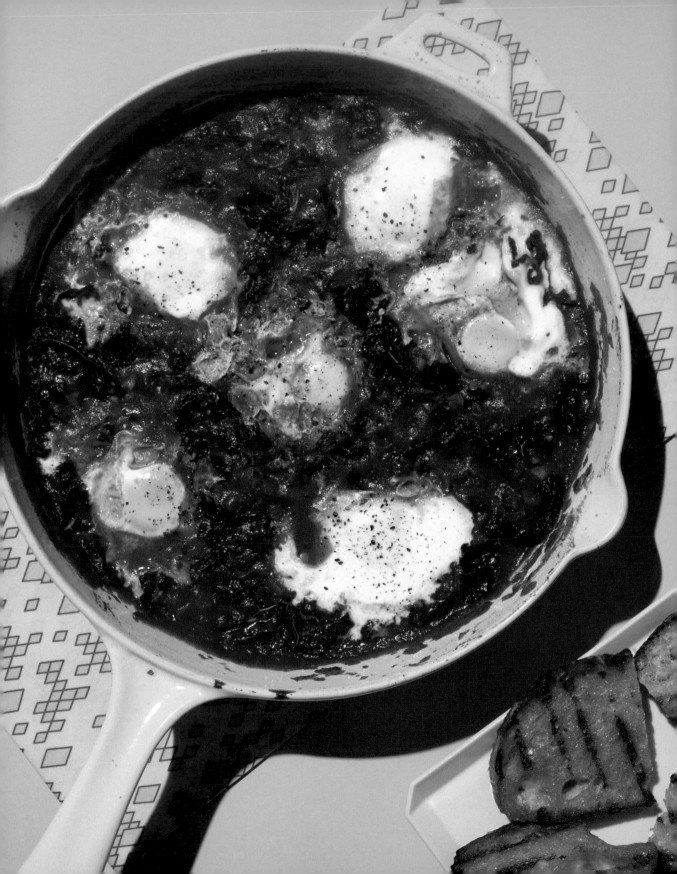

Spiced Kale Shakshuka

Serves 6

If cinnamon seems like a strange component to add to a tomato sauce, JUST TRUST US. You'll love it. If you don't like spicy, halve the amount of red pepper.

1. In a 12-inch skillet, combine 2 tablespoons of the olive oil, the crushed red pepper, and garlic and cook over medium heat for 2 minutes. Don't allow the garlic to brown.
2. Add the kale and a pinch of salt and sauté until it wilts, about 2 minutes. Transfer everything to a bowl and set aside.
3. In the same skillet, heat the remaining 2 tablespoons of the olive oil. Add the onion, season with a pinch of salt, and cook, stirring frequently, until the onion is fragrant and has softened, 3 to 4 minutes.
4. Stir in the cumin and cinnamon. Add the crushed tomatoes and 1 cup of water. Bring to a boil, then reduce the heat to low and cook until thickened, about 10 minutes. Season with salt to taste and stir in the sautéed kale.
5. Make 6 little wells in the sauce with the back of a spoon and crack an egg into each well. Cover the skillet and cook the eggs until the whites are cooked through and opaque, about 4 minutes—no peeking!
6. While the eggs are cooking, toast the bread and drizzle with some olive oil. Season the shakshuka with pepper and serve with the toast.

4 tablespoons extra virgin olive oil, plus more for drizzling
1 tablespoon crushed red pepper
2 garlic cloves, minced
1 bunch of kale, tough ribs removed, leaves chopped into bite-size pieces
Kosher salt
1 large yellow onion, diced
1 teaspoon ground cumin
¼ teaspoon ground cinnamon
1 (28-ounce) can crushed tomatoes
6 large eggs
6 thick slices country bread
Freshly ground pepper

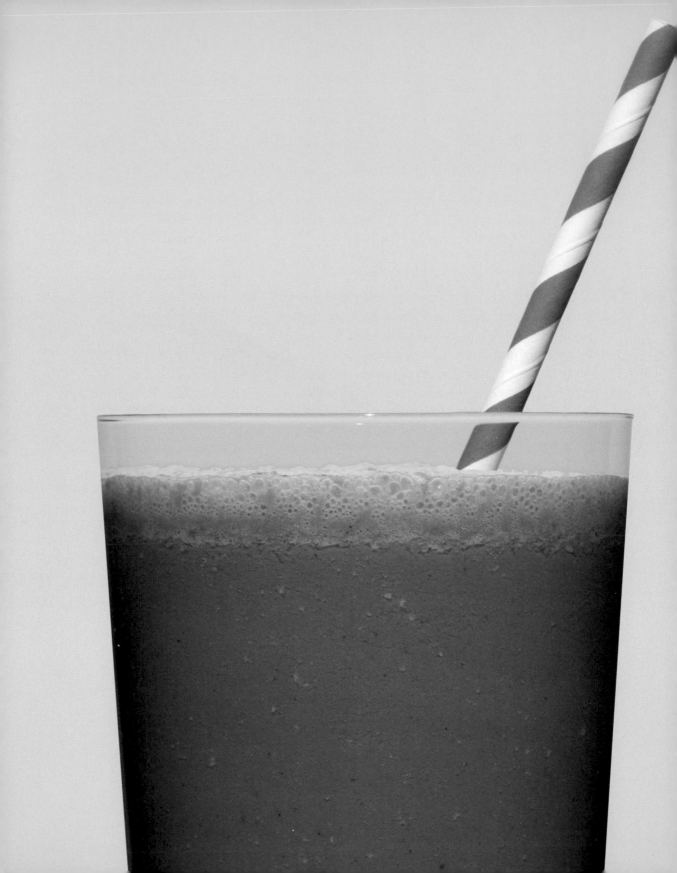

Elettra's Kale Smoothie
That Doesn't Taste Green

Makes 1 smoothie

I don't enjoy green drinks at all, but this is one smoothie I have developed for myself that I think tastes great AND has a good dose of raw greens. I drink this after my workouts and I am convinced it helps me to stay cold free throughout the winter. Any kind of green kale will do here, I just like lacinato the best. Also, if you're a dude, you can cut the Barlean's oil without it affecting the taste or consistency of the smoothie.

In a powerful blender, combine the whey protein, collagen, probiotics, yogurt, kale, coconut water, Barlean's oil (if using), and ice and blend until very smooth. Let the blender run for an extra 20 to 30 seconds more than you think it needs to really chop up the kale. If it's too thick for your liking, add ¼ to ½ cup water and blend again to combine. Enjoy immediately.

1 scoop (about ⅓ packed cup) vanilla whey protein (I use Bluebonnet)

1 tablespoon powdered collagen

1 serving powdered probiotics (usually ½ teaspoon)

¾ cup vegan coconut yogurt or full-fat Greek yogurt

4 cups kale, tough ribs and stems removed, leaves ripped into small pieces

1 cup raw coconut water or water

1 tablespoon Barlean's The Essential Woman oil (optional)

Small handful of ice

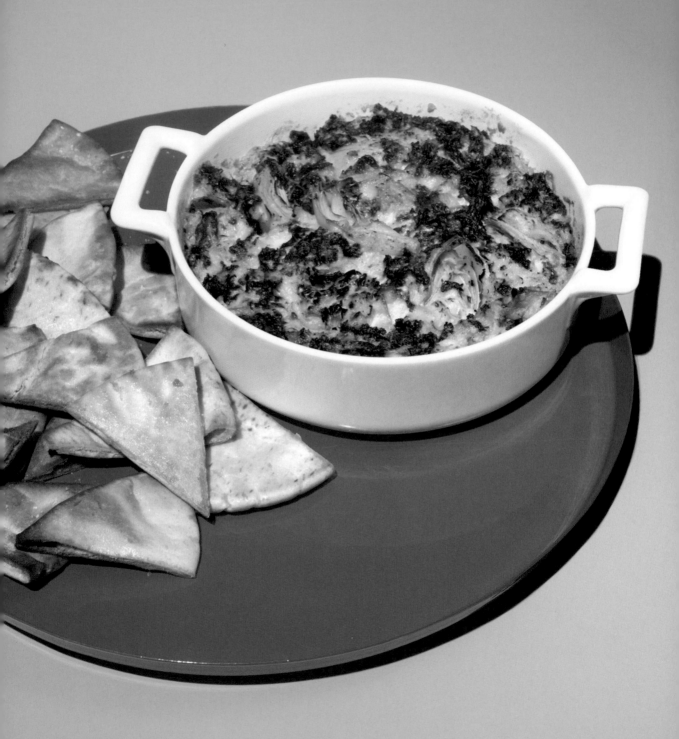

Kale Artichoke Dip

Serves 8 to 10

This dip will turn even the most intense kale skeptic into a believer. It can be served with toasted bread, warm pita bread, or chips.

1. Preheat the oven to 350°F. Butter a 10 x 6-inch baking dish.
2. In a 12-inch skillet, heat the olive oil over medium heat. Add the kale and a pinch of salt and sauté until it wilts, about 2 minutes. Transfer to a medium bowl and set aside.
3. In a food processor, combine the beans, garlic, and mayonnaise and puree until smooth.
4. Transfer the bean puree to a large bowl. Mix in the artichokes, kale, cheddar, 1 teaspoon of salt, and a few turns of pepper. Mix well to combine.
5. Spread the mixture into the buttered baking dish and bake for 30 minutes. If you want a browned top, place the baking dish under the broiler for 3 to 5 minutes.

Butter, for the baking dish
2 tablespoons extra virgin olive oil
1 bunch of kale, tough ribs and stems removed, roughly sliced into ½-inch-wide strips
Kosher salt
1 (15.5-ounce) can white beans, drained and rinsed
2 garlic cloves, peeled
½ cup mayonnaise
2 (6.5-ounce) jars marinated artichokes, drained and chopped
1 cup grated white cheddar cheese
Freshly ground pepper

One-Pot Lemony Kale and Quinoa Bowl

Serves 4 to 6

1 sweet potato, peeled and cut
    into ¼-inch cubes
4 cups low-sodium chicken stock
    or water
Kosher salt
2 cups quinoa
1 bunch of lacinato kale, tough
    ribs and stems removed, finely
    chopped
1 lemon, zested and juiced
8 tablespoons hummus
½ cup crumbled goat cheese
½ cup roasted almonds, chopped
Freshly ground pepper
Extra virgin olive oil

There are so many kinds of kale and I think most are interchangeable. I tend toward lacinato kale, because I find it to be the most flavorful and easiest to cook with, but if you prefer curly kale, or red Russian kale, or that's all you can find at your local market, those will work too. If you're a vegan, you can skip the goat cheese altogether—the hummus will do the work to provide some satisfying creaminess. This is also delicious with a spoonful of my vegan pesto (p. 60).

1. In a large pot, combine the sweet potato, chicken stock, and salt. Cover and bring to a boil.
2. Add the quinoa to the boiling stock and stir. Reduce the heat to a simmer, cover, and cook for 20 minutes—set a timer.
3. After 20 minutes, add the kale and lemon zest and stir a couple times. Remove from the heat, cover the pot, and allow everything to steam for 5 minutes—no peeking!
4. Mix in the lemon juice, then spoon the quinoa mixture into bowls. Top each serving with some hummus and sprinkle on the goat cheese, almonds, pepper, and a drizzle of olive oil. Enjoy!

LEEKS

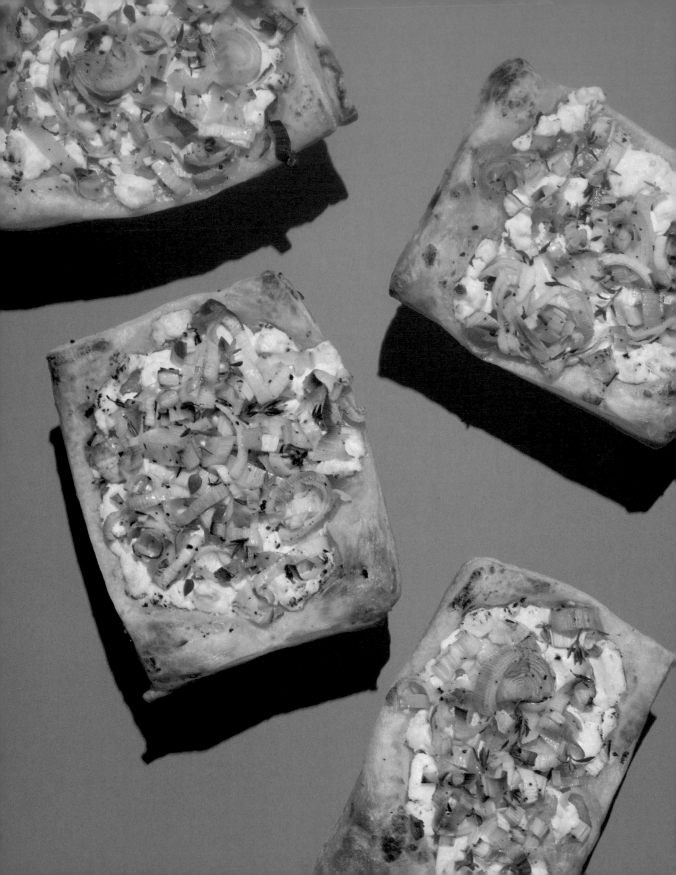

Leek Tartlets

Serves 6

Puff pastry always has to be thawed, which is not exactly impatient friendly—but planning ahead a little bit is totally worth it for these highly addictive and supereasy cheesy leek treats.

1. Preheat the oven to 375°F. Line a 15 x 10-inch baking sheet with parchment paper.
2. Cut the pastry dough into 6 rectangles and place on the baking sheet.
3. Sprinkle 2 tablespoons of the goat cheese onto each piece, leaving a ½-inch border all around.
4. In a bowl, combine the leeks, olive oil, thyme, and a generous pinch of salt and pepper. Toss to combine.
5. Top each rectangle with a small handful (about ¼ cup) of the leek mixture.
6. Bake until the dough is golden brown and puffed up, about 30 minutes. Allow to cool for a few minutes. Add some more pepper, if desired, and enjoy!

1 (14-ounce) box puff pastry (we like Dufour's Classic), thawed
12 tablespoons crumbled goat cheese
2 large leeks, white and light green parts only, cleaned, halved lengthwise, and sliced into half-moons
2 tablespoons extra virgin olive oil
1 tablespoon fresh thyme leaves
Kosher salt and freshly ground pepper

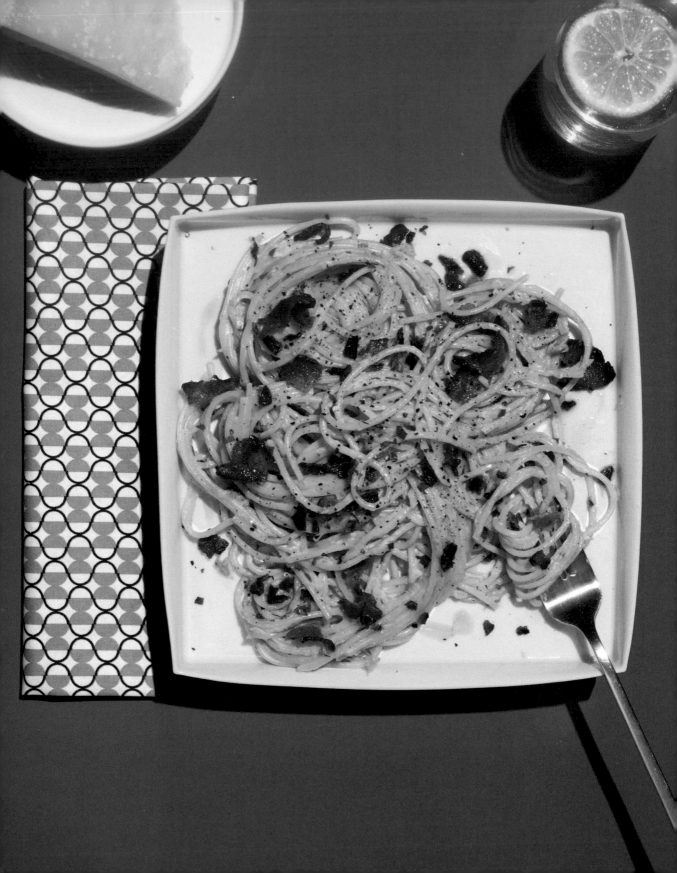

Melt-in-Your-Mouth Leeks Carbonara

Serves 4 to 6

This is a recipe where getting your mise en place together before you start is especially important! Once the spaghetti is done cooking and drained, you have to work fast.

Kosher salt

8 slices bacon

3 leeks, white and light green parts only, cleaned and cut into ¼-inch slices

1 lemon, zested and juiced

Extra virgin olive oil

3 large eggs

½ cup grated Parmigiano-Reggiano cheese, plus a small handful for garnish

½ cup chopped fresh flat leaf parsley

Freshly ground pepper

1 pound spaghetti

1. Bring a large pot of salted water to a boil.
2. In a large pan or skillet, cook the bacon over medium-high heat until very crispy, about 10 minutes. Drain on a paper towel. Reserve 2 to 3 tablespoons of bacon fat and discard the remainder.
3. Return the reserved bacon fat to the pan and cook the leeks until they are very soft, 10 to 15 minutes. Make sure to stir them frequently so that they do not burn. Transfer the leeks to a food processor, add the lemon juice, and pulse until the leeks turn into a smooth paste. If you need to loosen the mixture in the food processor, you can add a little bit of olive oil (about 1 tablespoon total). Let the leeks cool in the food processor while you make the egg mixture.
4. In a large serving bowl, whisk the eggs, Parmigiano, parsley, lemon zest, and a generous pinch of salt and pepper. Add the leeks to the egg mixture a little at a time and stir with each addition. (If the leeks are too hot they'll cook the eggs, which you don't want, so really wait until the leeks have cooled down.)
5. Add the spaghetti to the boiling water and cook according to the package directions. Reserving ¼ cup of the pasta cooking water, drain the spaghetti and very quickly add it to the large bowl with the egg mixture—the heat from the spaghetti will cook the eggs.
6. If the spaghetti looks dry, add in the reserved cooking water, a little bit at a time, and mix until you reach a desired consistency. Crumble the bacon and toss to combine. Top with a drizzle of olive oil and extra Parmigiano.

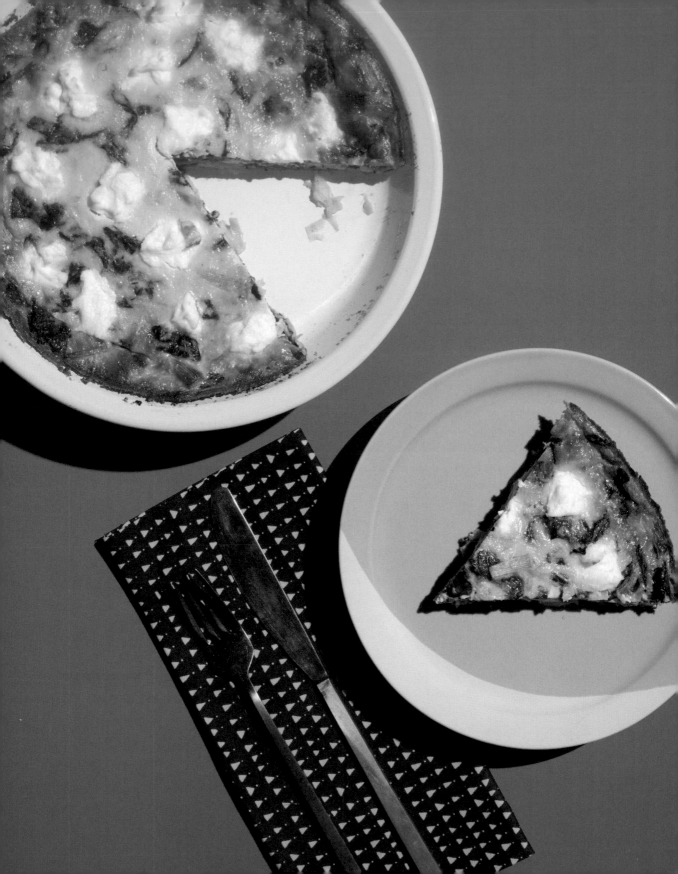

Leek and Spinach Quiche

Serves 6 to 8

The baking time on this is a little on the longer side, but the prep is quick and easy. You could make this on a Sunday when you have a little more time to devote to cooking, and use the leftovers as meals for the rest of the week!

1. Preheat the oven to 350°F. Coat a pie pan with cooking spray.
2. Make the bread crumb crust: Scatter the bread crumbs evenly in the pie pan. Shake the pan gently to distribute the crumbs all over the sides and bottom. Wipe excess crumbs off the outer edge of the pan and sprinkle the Asiago over the bottom. Set aside.
3. In a large pot, melt the butter over medium heat. Add the leeks and garlic and cook, stirring frequently, until the leeks are softened, about 5 minutes.
4. Add the spinach and nutmeg and cook until the spinach is fully wilted and any liquid evaporates, about 4 minutes. Transfer to a bowl and let cool a bit. Pop the mixture in the freezer if you're impatient!
5. In a separate large bowl, combine the eggs, heavy cream, and a generous pinch of salt and pepper. Whisk together until frothy and then add in the leek mixture and stir to combine.
6. Pour the contents of the bowl into the prepared pie pan. Add the ricotta in small dollops over the top and sprinkle with the Asiago.
7. Bake until the center of the quiche is set and the cheese starts to brown, 40 to 45 minutes. Let cool for about 20 minutes before serving. Quiche is also excellent served cold or at room temperature.

BREAD CRUMB CRUST

2 tablespoons unseasoned dried bread crumbs

¼ cup grated Asiago or Gruyère cheese, grated on a rasp-style zester

QUICHE FILLING

2 tablespoons unsalted butter

2 medium leeks, white and light green parts only, cleaned and quartered lengthwise, and chopped roughly (will yield about 2 cups)

2 garlic cloves, minced

3 cups packed spinach

1 teaspoon ground nutmeg

4 large eggs

¾ cup heavy cream

Kosher salt and freshly ground pepper

¼ cup whole-milk ricotta cheese

¼ cup grated Asiago or Gruyère cheese

Leek Butter

Makes ½ cup

2 leeks, white and light green
    parts only, cleaned and halved
    lengthwise
½ cup low-sodium chicken stock
Kosher salt and freshly ground
    pepper
4 tablespoons (½ stick) unsalted
    butter, at room temperature
Zest of ½ lemon
½ tablespoon finely chopped
    fresh chives

This multi-use butter works on everything from toast with fried egg, to pasta, to chicken and fish. The recipe yields quite a bit of butter, so store whatever you're not going to use in the following week in the freezer in ice cube trays.

1. In a skillet, lay the leeks in a single layer and pour in the chicken stock, so that the liquid comes halfway up the leeks (add water, if more liquid is needed). Season with 2 pinches of salt and several turns of pepper. Bring to a boil over high heat, then reduce to a simmer, cover, and cook until very soft, 15 to 20 minutes.
2. Drain the leeks and allow them to cool in a colander in the sink. Once cooled, transfer them to a food processor with the softened butter and process until smooth, about 30 seconds.
3. Transfer the butter to a small bowl and stir in the lemon zest, chives, and 2 pinches of salt. Stir to combine with a spatula.
4. Store in a jar, ramekin, or food storage container. Refrigerate until hardened. It can be stored in the fridge for up to 1 week, or freeze it in an ice cube tray for up to 6 months.

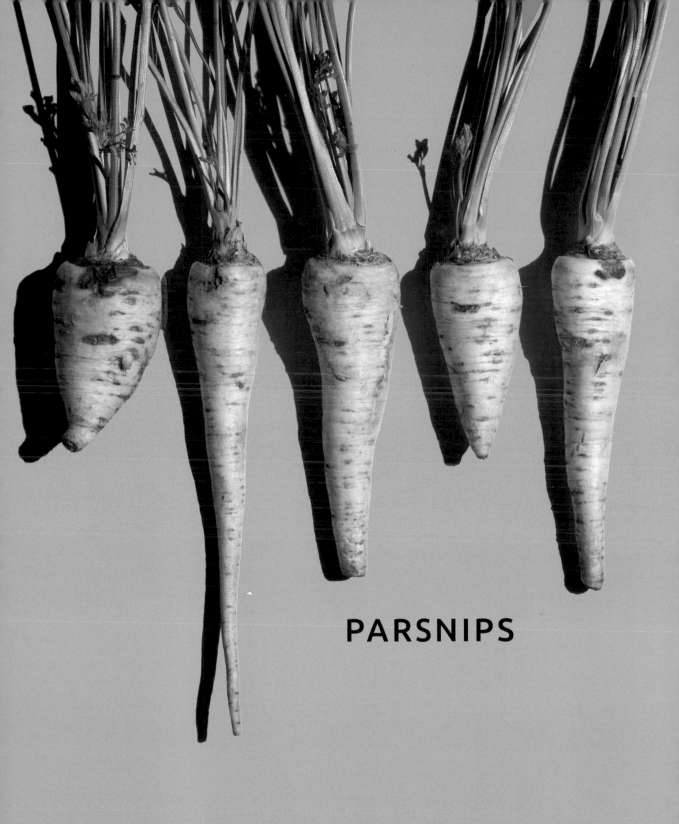

PARSNIPS

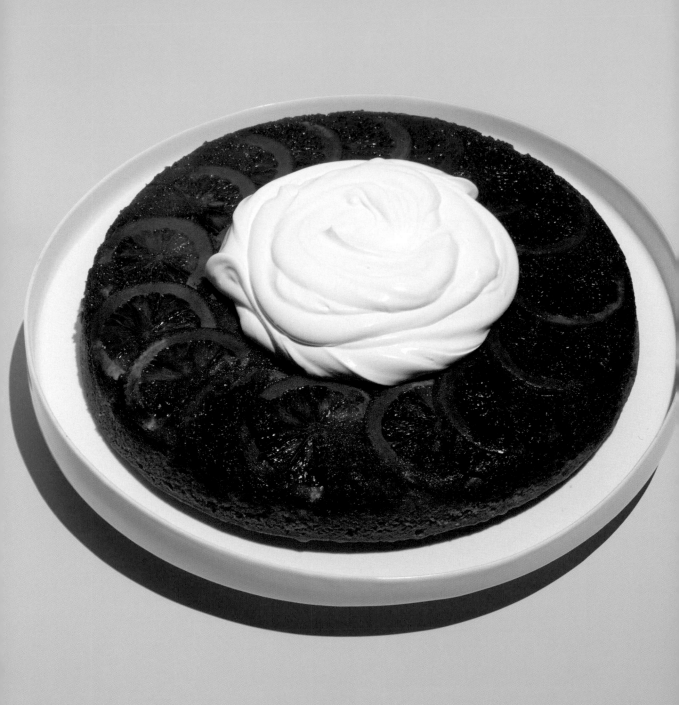

Upside-Down Blood Orange Parsnip Cake

Serves 6 to 8

Parsnips in a cake?! Yep. And you'll be blown away by how delicious this is. The vanilla cake mix does a lot of the heavy lifting here as far as measuring things out and making a mess (and more dishes). In this cake recipe, the eggs, oil, and water needed for preparing the batter are listed in the ingredients below because the amounts differ slightly from the box directions. Also, if you can't find blood oranges, regular oranges will work too.

6 tablespoons sugar

2 tablespoons unsalted butter

3 blood oranges, thinly sliced

1 (15.25-ounce) box vanilla cake mix

1 tablespoon ground cinnamon

2 large eggs

½ cup extra virgin olive oil

1 medium to large parsnip, peeled and grated (should yield about 1 cup)

1 vanilla bean, sliced open lengthwise

Whipped cream, for garnish (optional)

1. Preheat the oven to 350°F.
2. In a 12-inch ovenproof skillet, dissolve the sugar in 3 tablespoons of water over medium heat. Bring to a boil and cook for 4 minutes, not stirring, until the syrup is darkened.
3. Remove from the heat and whisk in the butter. Lay the blood orange slices in the pan, overlapping slightly. Coat the sides of the pan with cooking spray. Set aside.
4. Make the cake batter by combining the dry cake mix, cinnamon, eggs, olive oil, 1 cup water, and the parsnips. Scrape the vanilla seeds out of the bean into the batter. Whisk to combine well.
5. Pour the batter over the blood oranges and spread evenly with a spatula. Bake until a toothpick comes out clean and the cake is golden brown, 30 to 35 minutes.
6. Let the cake cool completely in the pan. Invert a large dish over the skillet and swiftly (and gracefully!) flip the skillet over to bring the blood orange to the top of the cake. Serve and enjoy with a dollop of whipped cream, if desired.

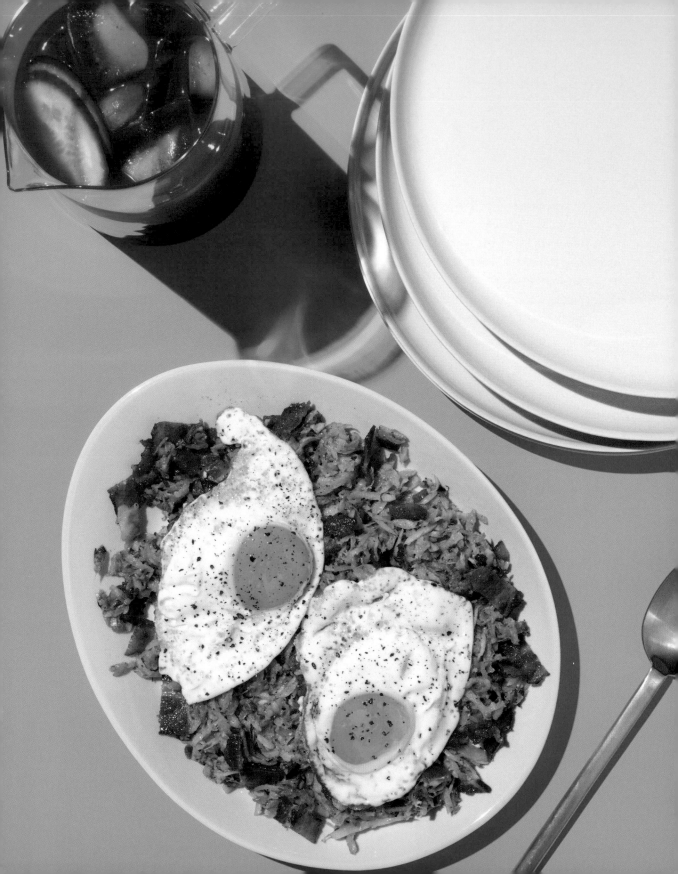

Parsnip Bacon Hash

Serves 4 to 6

This parsnip hash would be excellent with a fried egg on top. It also keeps beautifully in the fridge so it can be used as part of breakfast throughout the week. If you're making this hash for a weekend brunch, may I recommend you pair it with an Impatient Bloody Mary (page 128).

1. In a large bowl, combine the grated parsnips, onion, lemon juice, sage, Parmigiano, and a generous pinch of salt, and stir to combine. Set aside.
2. In a large skillet, cook the bacon over medium-high heat until crispy, about 4 minutes on both sides. Drain the bacon on paper towels.
3. Pour the excess bacon fat out of the skillet into a small bowl. Then transfer 2 tablespoons of the bacon fat back into the skillet along with the butter. Allow the butter to melt over medium heat, then add the parsnip mix. Cook for about 10 minutes, stirring frequently, until the parsnip hash is golden brown.
4. Crumble the bacon and add it into the parsnip hash. Stir to combine and enjoy.

3 parsnips, peeled and grated on the large teardrops of a box grater
1 small yellow onion, grated on the large teardrops of a box grater
1 lemon, juiced
¼ cup fresh sage leaves, minced
½ cup grated Parmigiano-Reggiano cheese
Kosher salt
10 slices bacon
1 tablespoon unsalted butter

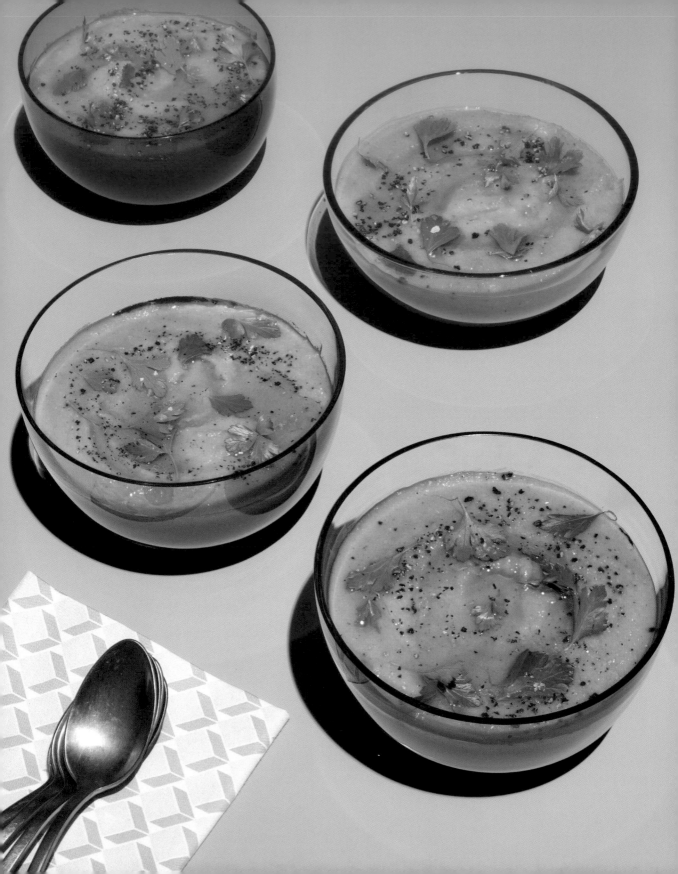

Hearty Parsnip Soup

Serves 4 to 6

I know the ingredient list here looks intimidating, but you don't have to chop anything perfectly. It's all going to simmer and soften in a pot and get blitzed into a lovely, hearty puree.

1. In a large pot, heat the olive oil. Add the turmeric, rosemary, tarragon, garlic, and onion and cook, stirring occasionally, until the onion is softened and translucent, about 5 minutes. Season with a generous pinch of salt and pepper.
2. Add the sweet potato, fennel, and parsnips and cook, stirring frequently, for an additional 5 minutes.
3. Add the wine and scrape the sides and bottom of the pot (this is called "deglazing"—you fancy!). Let the wine reduce about 5 minutes, stirring occasionally.
4. Add the stock and bring to a boil. Reduce the heat to low, cover, and cook for 15 to 20 minutes, until the vegetables have softened.
5. Remove from the heat, add the sesame oil and lemon juice, and puree with an immersion blender or regular blender until completely smooth. Taste and add more salt and pepper, if desired. Serve each bowl with a drizzle of olive oil and a sprinkle of parsley.

2 tablespoons extra virgin olive oil, plus more for drizzling
½ teaspoon ground turmeric
2 tablespoons chopped fresh rosemary
2 tablespoons chopped fresh tarragon
3 garlic cloves, sliced
1 medium yellow onion, chopped
Kosher salt and freshly ground pepper
1 sweet potato, peeled and chopped
1 bulb fennel (stalks, fronds, and outer leaves discarded), bulb chopped
4 parsnips, peeled and chopped
1 cup white wine
4 cups low-sodium vegetable or chicken stock
2 tablespoons toasted sesame oil
2 lemons, juiced
4 tablespoons minced fresh flat leaf parsley, for garnish

Parsnip Fries with Grainy Mustard–Mayo Dip

Serves 4 to 6

4 parsnips, peeled and cut into fry
    shapes (see headnote)
3 tablespoons extra virgin olive oil
2 garlic cloves, minced
1 tablespoon finely chopped fresh
    rosemary
1 tablespoon fresh thyme
Kosher salt and freshly ground
    pepper

MUSTARD-MAYO DIP
¼ cup mayonnaise
1 tablespoon grainy mustard
1 tablespoon Dijon mustard
1 tablespoon honey
Kosher salt and freshly ground
    pepper

Parsnips are often awkwardly shaped for cutting. The best way to cut one into a fry shape is to trim the narrow end and then halve the thicker part of the parsnip and cut the fry shapes from there. Use the narrow end in your parsnip cake or soup (pages 79 and 83).

1. Preheat the oven to 400°F. Line a 15 x 10-inch baking sheet with parchment paper.
2. In a large bowl, toss together the parsnips, olive oil, garlic, rosemary, thyme, and a generous pinch of salt and pepper.
3. Lay the parsnip fries onto the baking sheet, being careful not to let them overlap. Bake for 10 minutes. Gently shake the pan to toss them around and bake until golden brown and tender, another 10 minutes.
4. Meanwhile, make the dip: In a small bowl, stir together the mayonnaise, grainy mustard, Dijon mustard, honey, and a small pinch of salt and pepper.
5. Transfer the fries to a serving dish. Serve with the mustard-mayo dip.

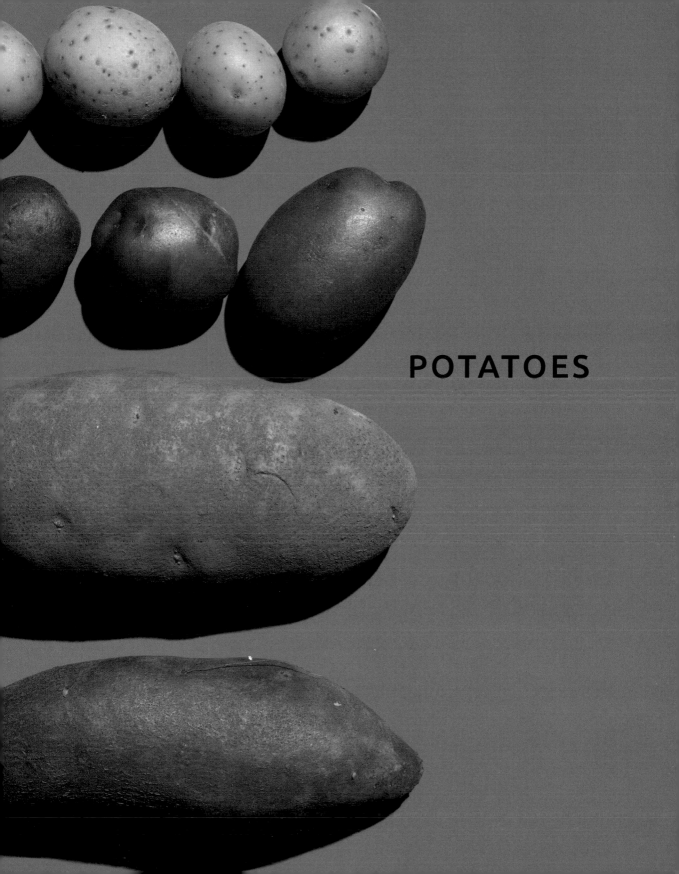

POTATOES

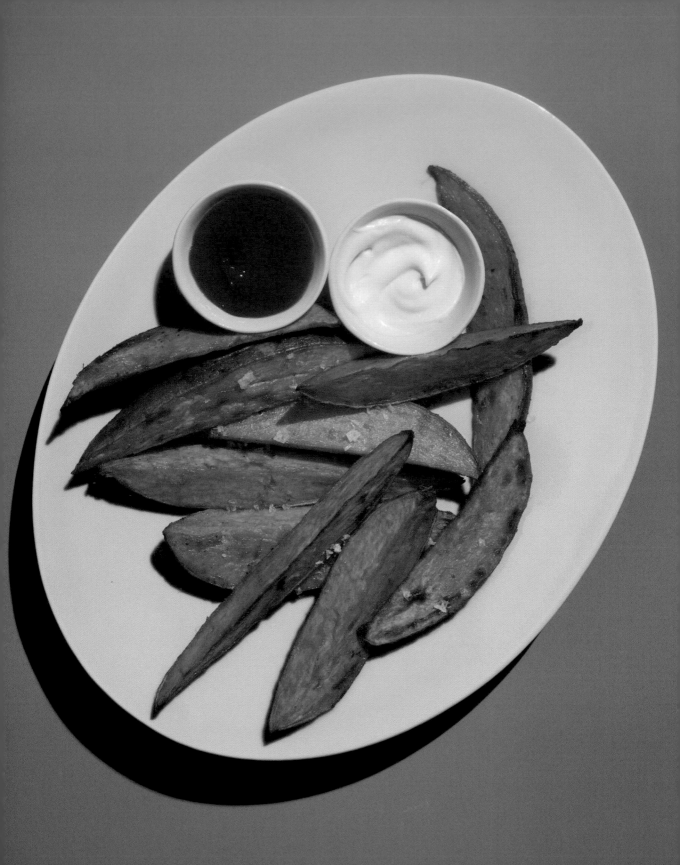

Baked Yam Sriracha Wedges

Serves 4 to 6

Whenever I have extra yams, I love making these fries. They are great as a side or even wrapped up in a tortilla with a fried egg, avocado, fresh greens, and drizzled with Sriracha. You can also sub in sweet potatoes.

3 small yams, sliced into wedges
4 tablespoons extra virgin olive oil
2 tablespoons Sriracha sauce
Kosher salt
Condiment of your choice

1. Preheat the oven to 450°F. Line a 15 x 10-inch baking sheet with parchment paper or foil.
2. In a large bowl, combine the yam wedges, olive oil, Sriracha, and 2 generous pinches of salt. Use tongs to combine well.
3. Place the wedges on the baking sheet, keeping about 1 inch between them. Bake for 15 minutes, then flip the wedges and bake until the wedges are tender when pierced with a fork, another 10 to 15 minutes.
4. Serve immediately with the condiment of your choice (I personally love these dipped in mayonnaise . . . then again, I love almost anything in mayonnaise).

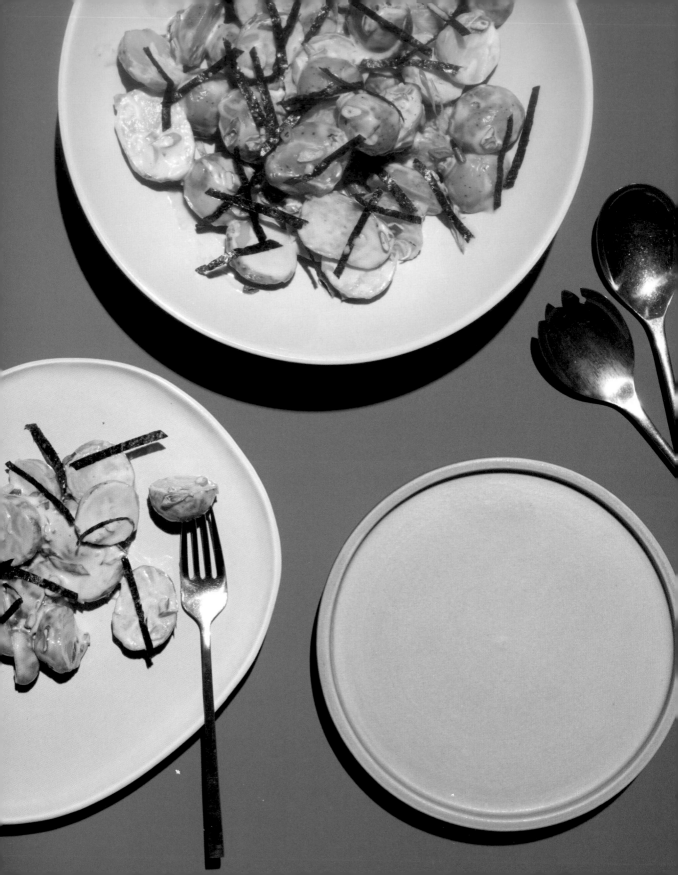

Miso Potato Salad with Crunchy Sesame Seaweed

Serves 4 to 6

My memories of potato salad are not great: I think of the ubiquitous supermushy, mayo-drowned heaps from local NYC delis I grew up with. But here we put a flavor twist on potato salad, using seaweed snacks and miso, which makes it totally irresistible.

3 pounds baby potatoes
½ cup mayonnaise
4 tablespoons white miso paste
¼ cup ume plum vinegar
1 heaping teaspoon kosher salt
2 tablespoons honey
2 bunches of scallions, thinly sliced
1 (0.35-ounce) package roasted sesame seaweed snack, cut into thin strips

1. Place the baby potatoes in a large pot, cover with cold water, and bring to a boil over high heat. Cook until tender, 10 to 12 minutes.
2. Meanwhile, in a small bowl, whisk together the mayonnaise, miso, vinegar, salt, and honey.
3. Drain the potatoes well, then put them back in the same pot to evaporate any remaining water. When cool enough to handle, cut the potatoes in half.
4. Add the mayo mixture and stir well to combine. Add the scallions and seaweed strips. Taste and add more salt, if desired.

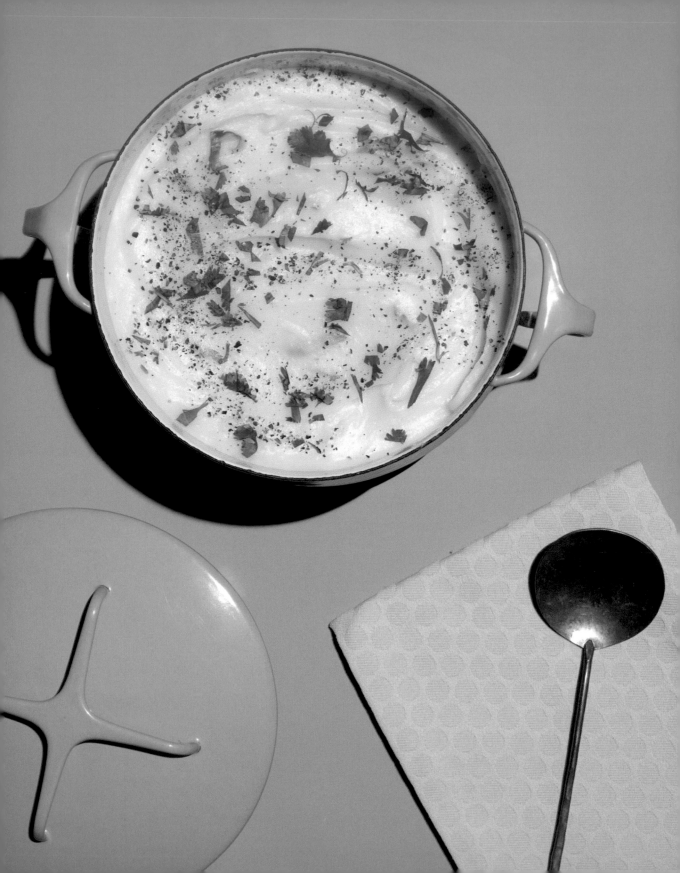

Coconut-Cilantro Mashed Potatoes

Serves 4 to 6

I never thought of mashed potatoes as that exciting, but with a little coconut milk and cilantro you can turn them into something unexpected and comforting.

2 pounds russet potatoes (about 4 medium), peeled and chopped
Kosher salt
1 (13.5-ounce) can unsweetened coconut milk
Freshly ground pepper
¼ cup minced fresh cilantro

1. Place the potatoes in a large pot and add the coconut milk and a generous pinch of salt. Bring to a boil over high heat, then reduce the heat to low, cover, and cook until the potatoes are easily pierced with a fork, 10 to 15 minutes.
2. With an immersion blender or regular blender, puree the potatoes until smooth, adding salt and pepper to taste. Be careful not to overpuree the potatoes, because they can become gummy.
3. Gently stir in the cilantro and serve immediately.

Surprise Potegg

Serves 4

4 small to medium russet potatoes
    (see headnote)
4 tablespoons (½ stick) unsalted
    butter, cut into 8 slices
Kosher salt
1 teaspoon distilled white vinegar
4 large eggs
½ cup sour cream
¼ cup chopped fresh flat leaf
    parsley, for garnish

I'll admit that this recipe is a little ridiculous, but it holds a special place in my heart because it was one of the first I developed for *Impatient Foodie*. The inspiration for it came from a story about a friend of mine who went to a superfancy dinner party, only to be served a seemingly simple, sad baked potato. When he cut into the potato, a perfectly poached egg came oozing out, followed by the waiters lifting covers off of some bowls on the dinner table to reveal an assortment of decadent toppings, including different types of caviar. I have made poteggs (minus the caviar) for a few friends and the look on their faces when an unexpected egg comes oozing out of their boring-looking baked potato is priceless. When choosing your potatoes, imagine that you'll be cutting out a circle on one side and scooping out a little bit of the potato flesh to nestle in your poached egg. The potato should be about twice the size of an egg, but not larger because that's a bad egg : potato ratio tastewise.

1. Preheat the oven to 425°F.
2. Cut 4 sheets of foil large enough to completely wrap the potatoes.
3. Wash the potatoes, dry well, and prick several times with a fork. Place each potato on a piece of foil with a slice of butter underneath and a slice of butter on top. Sprinkle with salt, and tightly seal each potato in the foil. Bake for 30 minutes, then flip the potatoes over, and bake for another 30 minutes. Test the potatoes for doneness by piercing them with a fork. Take the potatoes out, but leave the oven on and reduce the temperature to 250°F.
4. When the potatoes are cool enough to handle, unwrap them and cut out a circular well at the top of each potato to hold

the poached egg, taking care not to cut through the bottom of the potato. Reserve the skin that you cut out (you will be using it as a lid later). Transfer the potatoes to the oven to keep them warm while you poach the eggs.

5. Fill a saucepan with about 2 inches of water and add the vinegar. Bring to a boil over medium-high heat. When the water starts to boil, reduce the heat to a simmer. Crack each egg into a small bowl (4 separate bowls). With a spoon, gently swirl the boiling water around the perimeter of the pan to create a small whirlpool. Gently pour the eggs into the center of the whirlpool, one at a time, and let them cook for 3½ minutes. With a slotted spoon, remove the eggs from the water and drain on paper towels.

6. Remove the potatoes from the oven and gently place a poached egg inside the hole, trimming excess egg white to fit inside the potato well, if necessary. Cover the egg with the reserved potato skin to hide it, then cover the incision area with sour cream and parsley. Enjoy immediately.

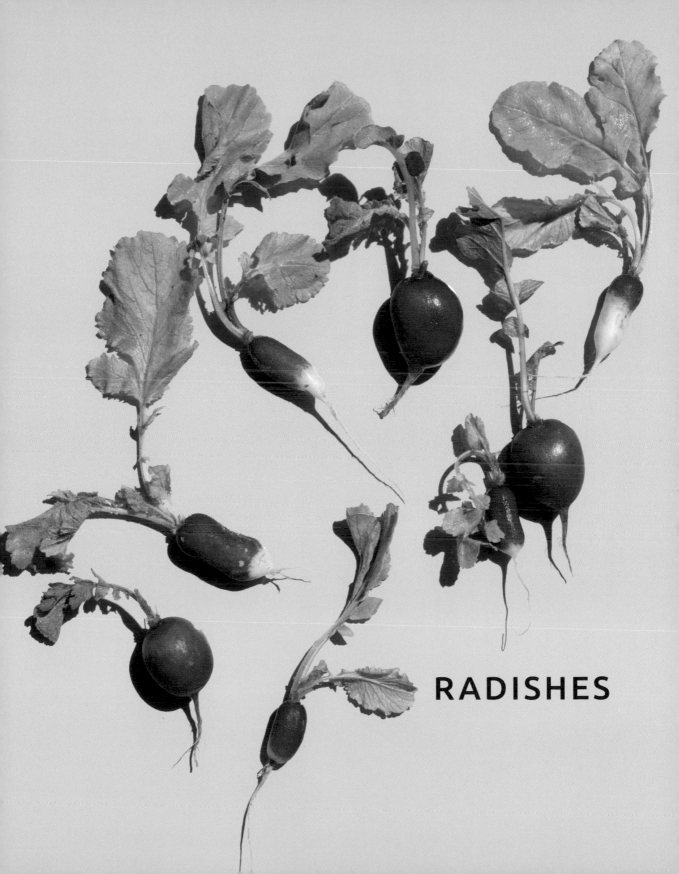

RADISHES

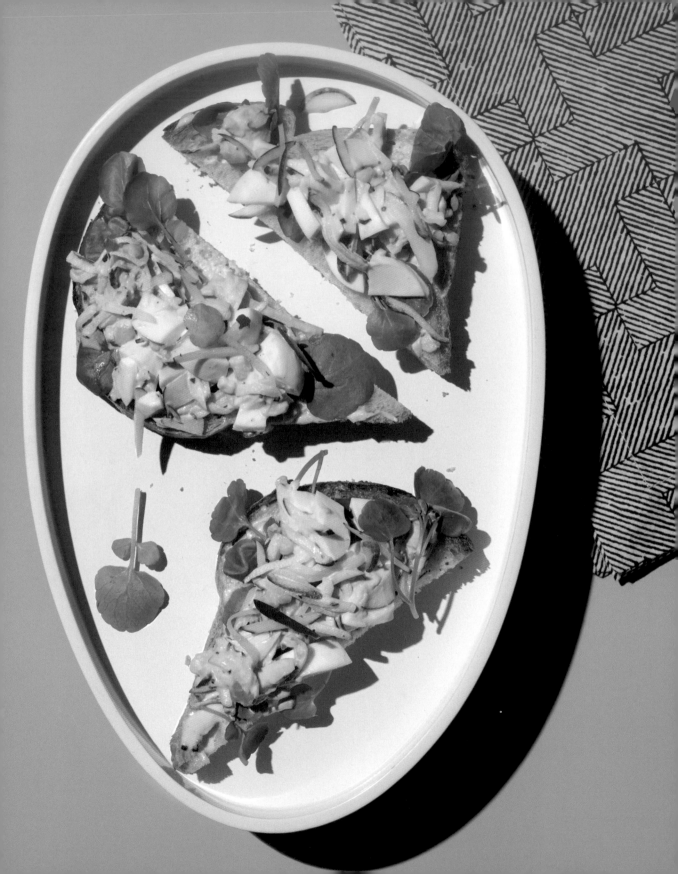

Radish Egg Salad

Serves 4 to 6

This fresh and light radish egg salad can be enjoyed on its own, or served as a salad on a bed of watercress, or on a slice of toasted bread with scattered watercress as an open-faced sandwich.

6 large eggs

⅓ cup mayonnaise

1 teaspoon toasted sesame oil

½ teaspoon mirin

2 teaspoons rice vinegar

Kosher salt and freshly ground pepper

1 bunch of radishes, green tops removed, grated on the large teardrops of a box grater

1 bunch of watercress

1. Bring a medium pot of water to a boil. Gently drop in the eggs and set a timer for 10 minutes.
2. Meanwhile, in a small bowl, whisk together the mayonnaise, sesame oil, mirin, and rice vinegar. Taste and add salt and pepper to your liking.
3. When the eggs have cooked for 10 minutes, run them under very cold water. When cool enough to handle, peel the shells off.
4. Place the eggs in a medium bowl and coarsely mash them with a fork. Add the radishes and mayonnaise dressing and mix together well. Serve on a bed of watercress.

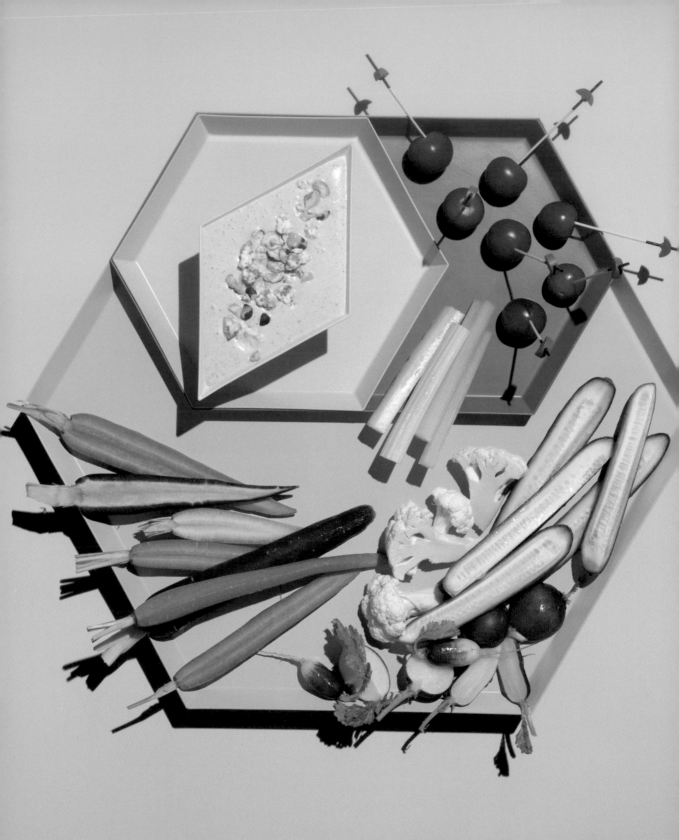

Radish Dip with Crudités

Serves 4 to 6

If you're not a huge fan of ranch dressing–type crudité dips, this radish dip is a great substitute. It is bold and bright in flavor while retaining the satiating thickness of store-bought dips.

½ cup raw hazelnuts, skinned or unskinned
1 bunch of radishes, green tops removed, chopped
1 (8-ounce) package cream cheese
1 lemon, zested, ½ juiced
Kosher salt
¼ cup crumbled blue cheese
2 tablespoons fresh flat leaf parsley leaves, minced, for garnish (optional)
Raw vegetables, for dipping

1. In a small pan, toast the hazelnuts over medium-high heat for about 3 minutes. Transfer them to a cutting board, chop coarsely, and set aside.
2. In a food processor, combine the radishes, cream cheese, lemon zest, lemon juice, and 2 generous pinches of salt and process until smooth.
3. Transfer the dip to a bowl and add the hazelnuts and blue cheese. Stir to combine and garnish with the parsley, if desired. Serve with the vegetables.

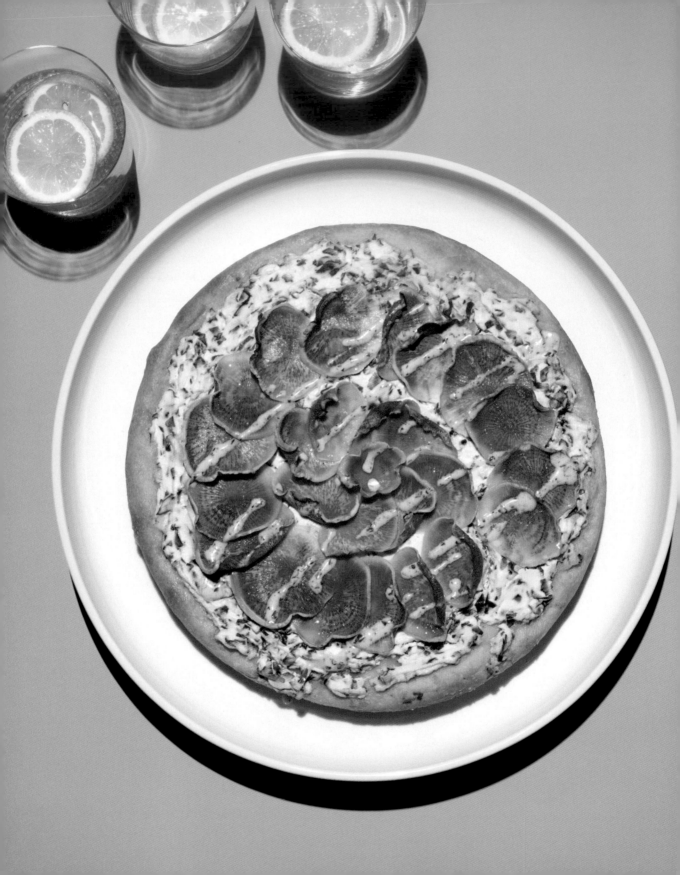

Watermelon Radish Pizza

Serves 4 to 6

Coming up with unique ideas for watermelon radishes posed a bit of a challenge. I believe there is an old adage that says, "When in doubt, make pizza." It worked like a charm.

1. Preheat the oven to 400°F. Grease an ovenproof skillet with 2 tablespoons of the olive oil.
2. Press the pizza dough over the bottom of the skillet to form a round. Brush the dough with olive oil and scatter a pinch of salt.
3. In a small bowl, combine the basil, ricotta, and a generous pinch of salt and pepper. Spread the ricotta mixture over the pizza dough, leaving a 1½-inch border all around.
4. Layer the sliced radishes over the ricotta mixture, slightly overlapping. Drizzle with a little olive oil. Bake until the pizza crust is golden brown, about 30 minutes. Check the pizza at the halfway point. Tent the radishes with foil if they brown before the crust.
5. Meanwhile, make the herbed mayonnaise: In a blender, combine the mayonnaise, lemon zest, lemon juice, parsley, and a pinch of salt and pepper and blend until the mayonnaise takes on a green tint from the parsley. Place the mixture in a zip-seal plastic bag and set aside.
6. Remove the pizza from the oven and allow to cool, about 5 minutes. Cut a tiny corner off the plastic bag and pipe the mayonnaise over the pizza. Slice and serve.

Extra virgin olive oil

1 pound store-bought pizza dough, refrigerated or thawed frozen

Kosher salt

2 cups fresh basil leaves, finely chopped

2 cups ricotta cheese

Freshly ground pepper

1 small to medium watermelon radish, peeled and sliced on a mandoline 1/16 inch thick

HERBED MAYONNAISE

½ cup mayonnaise

1 lemon, zested, ½ juiced

1 tablespoon fresh flat leaf parsley, chopped

Kosher salt and freshly ground pepper

Radish-Cucumber Gazpacho

Serves 4 to 6

2 cucumbers, peeled
½ avocado
½ cup extra virgin olive oil
1 bunch of radishes, green tops
    removed, chopped
1 garlic clove, peeled
½ small red onion, roughly
    chopped
¼ cup full-fat Greek yogurt
¼ cup packed fresh dill
2 lemons, juiced
2 tablespoons red wine vinegar
Kosher salt and freshly ground
    pepper
1 cup watercress leaves, for
    garnish

Very hot and humid summer weather tends to cut my appetite. That's when gazpacho—a cold, light, summery soup—comes in. This version is radish based instead of tomato based. It's crisp and refreshing; we couldn't get enough.

1. Halve the cucumbers lengthwise. Using a spoon, scoop out all the seeds and discard them. Chop the cucumber.
2. Scoop the avocado into a blender. Add the olive oil, radishes, cucumbers, garlic, onion, yogurt, dill, lemon juice, vinegar, and a generous pinch of salt and pepper and blend until smooth.
3. Transfer the soup to serving bowls and garnish each bowl with the watercress.

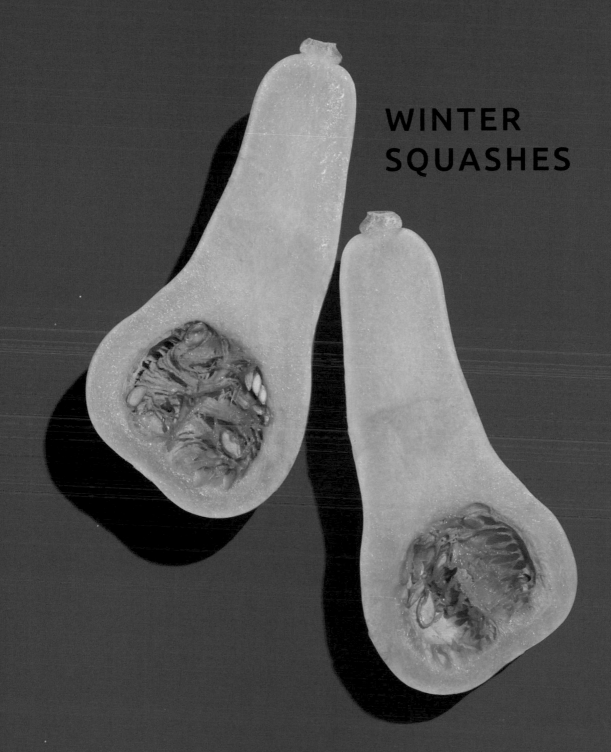

WINTER
SQUASHES

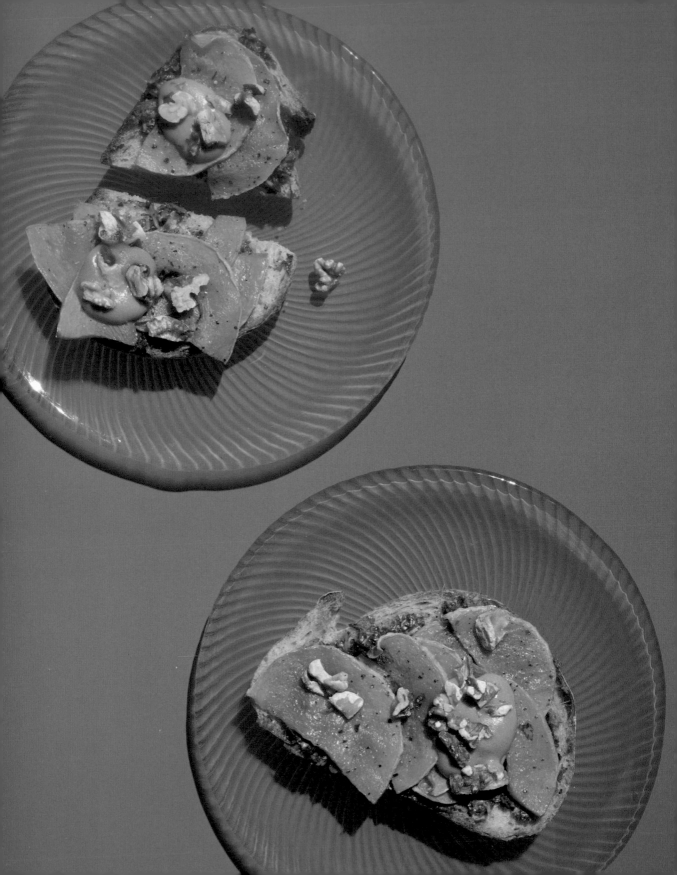

Butternut Squash Toasts

Serves 4

These toasts work nicely with Vegan Pesto (page 60) and the vinaigrette.

1. Preheat the oven to 400°F. Line a 15 x 10-inch baking sheet with parchment paper.
2. Place the butternut slices in a single layer on the baking sheet, drizzle with some olive oil, and sprinkle with a pinch of salt and pepper. Roast until the squash slices are very tender, 20 to 25 minutes.
3. Meanwhile, in a small bowl, whisk together the mustard and vinegar to make a paste. Then slowly whisk in 2 tablespoons of olive oil, a little at a time, to make a thick dressing. Add a pinch of salt. Set the vinaigrette aside.
4. Allow the butternut squash to cool for about 5 minutes. Smear the toast with pesto and top with the butternut squash, a small pinch of salt and pepper, a drizzle of the vinaigrette, and a sprinkle of the chopped walnuts.

1 medium butternut squash, peeled, halved lengthwise, seeded, and thinly sliced into ⅛-inch-thick half-rounds

Extra virgin olive oil

Kosher salt and freshly ground pepper

2 teaspoons Dijon mustard

1 teaspoon balsamic vinegar

4 slices bread, toasted

¼ cup Vegan Pesto (page 60), or store-bought

2 tablespoons chopped walnuts

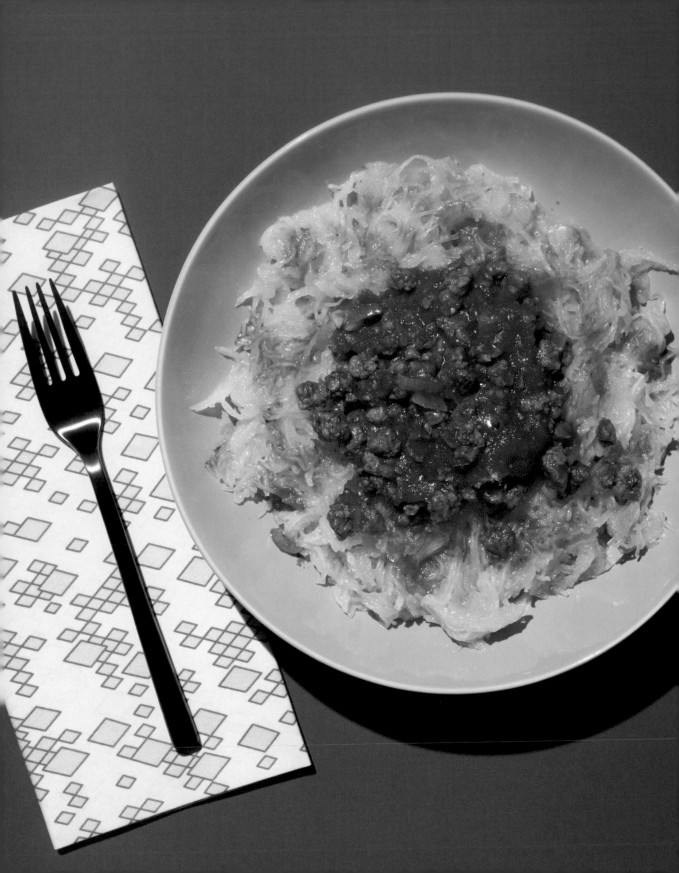

Spaghetti Squash Vegan "Bolognese"

Serves 4 to 6

I am not a vegan, but I do try to minimize the amount of meat and animal products I consume. Beyond Beef is a new plant protein beef substitute that I think tastes good, has a good texture, is easy to cook with, and doesn't hurt my stomach (unlike other meat substitutes I've tried in the past). I like their Beefy Crumble flavor for this recipe.

2 spaghetti squash

Extra virgin olive oil

Kosher salt and freshly ground pepper

2 garlic cloves, minced

1 medium yellow onion, chopped

½ cup red wine (optional)

1 (11-ounce) package Beyond Beef Crumble (Beefy Crumble) or 2 cups any ground beef substitute that you like

1 (28-ounce) can San Marzano whole tomatoes

¼ teaspoon ground nutmeg

½ cup shredded vegan cheese (your favorite) or, if you're not vegan, shredded Parmigiano-Reggiano cheese (optional)

¼ cup fresh basil, minced (optional)

1. Preheat the oven to 400°F. Line a 15 x 10-inch baking sheet with parchment paper or foil.
2. With a sharp knife, halve the spaghetti squashes lengthwise. Scoop out and discard the seeds. Rub the squash flesh with olive oil and sprinkle with salt and pepper.
3. Place the squash halves cut side down on the baking sheet and bake until you can easily pierce all the way through the flesh with a fork, 30 to 40 minutes.
4. Meanwhile, in a large skillet or saucepan, heat 3 tablespoons of olive oil over medium-high heat. Add the garlic and onion and cook until fragrant and the onion is translucent, 3 to 5 minutes. Stir in a generous pinch of salt and pepper.
5. Add the wine (if using) and allow to cook off for 2 to 3 minutes. Add the Beef Crumble and cook, stirring frequently, for 2 minutes.
6. Add the tomatoes (with their juice) and the nutmeg. Break up the tomatoes into chunks with a wooden spoon. Allow the sauce to start bubbling, then turn the heat down to a simmer. Cook, uncovered, until the liquid is evaporated and the sauce has thickened, about 20 minutes.
7. When the squashes are cooked, remove them from the oven, and allow them to cool down until they can be handled.

Flip them over and use a fork to scrape out the strands into a large bowl.

8. Add the tomato sauce and vegan cheese or Parmigiano (if using) and toss until the squash is evenly coated. If desired, garnish with the basil. Serve immediately.

Quick Kuri Squash Soup
with Bacon and Goat Cheese

Serves 4 to 6

This soup is thick and rich and perfect for those cold, rainy days when all you can do is cook and chill in front of Netflix.

1. In a large pot, cook the bacon over medium-high heat until it is browned and crispy, 4 to 5 minutes. Remove the bacon and set aside, leaving the bacon fat in the pot.
2. Add the chicken stock to the pot with two generous pinches of salt, and the kuri squash. Bring to a boil, then reduce the heat, cover, and cook until the squash is tender, about 15 minutes.
3. Reduce the heat to a simmer and use an immersion blender to puree the soup. Add the lemon juice and more salt to taste. Stir to combine. Throw in the spinach and stir until it just starts to wilt.
4. Transfer to serving bowls and garnish each with the goat cheese and a pinch of the bacon.

4 slices bacon, cut into 1-inch pieces
3 cups low-sodium chicken stock
Kosher salt
1 kuri squash, halved, seeded, and chopped into 2-inch pieces (no need to peel)
1 lemon, juiced
1 (8-ounce) container prewashed spinach
4 to 6 tablespoons goat cheese

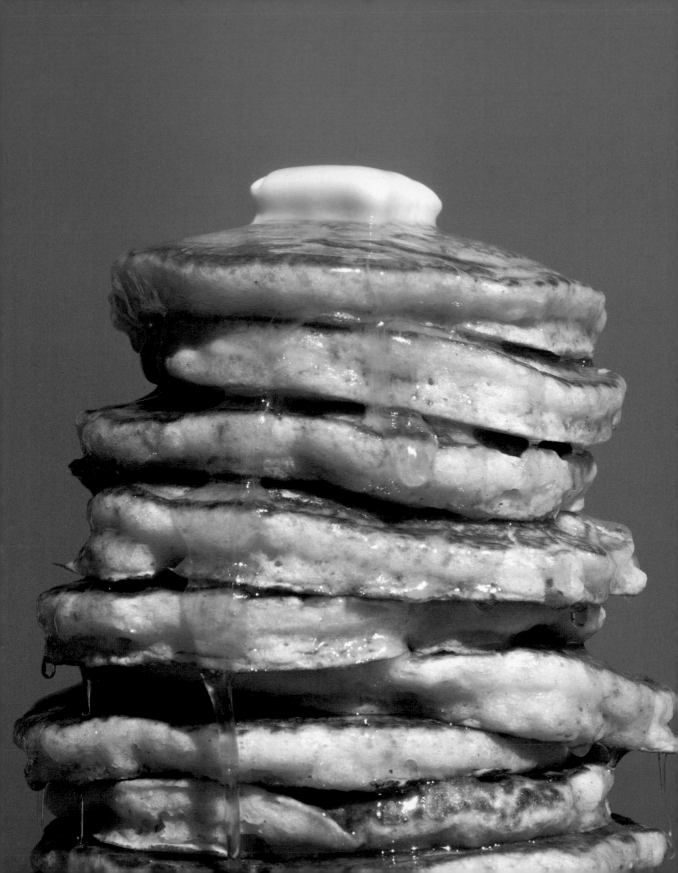

Acorn Squash Pancakes

Makes 10 to 12 pancakes

This recipe will yield double the amount of squash you need for 10 to 12 pancakes. Freeze the other half and reserve it for your next pancake craving—less work for the next batch!

1 acorn squash, halved and seeded
2 tablespoons extra virgin olive oil
¼ cup packed light brown sugar
1 heaping teaspoon ground cinnamon
¼ teaspoon kosher salt
2½ cups "just add water" pancake mix
¼ cup maple syrup, plus more for serving
4 tablespoons (½ stick) unsalted butter, plus more for serving

1. Preheat the oven to 400°F. Line a 15 x 10-inch baking sheet with foil.
2. Rub the acorn squash flesh with the olive oil and sprinkle evenly with the brown sugar, cinnamon, and salt. Place the halves on the baking sheet, cut side up, and bake until the squash flesh can be easily pierced with a fork, about 45 minutes.
3. When the squash is done baking, remove from the oven and allow to cool until you can handle. Scoop out the flesh of one half and put in a small bowl and mash well with a fork. (Reserve the other half for future use—see headnote.)
4. In a separate bowl, make the pancake batter according to the package directions, adding the maple syrup. Stir in the mashed squash to combine.
5. In a large skillet, melt 2 tablespoons of the butter over medium heat. Add ¼ cup of batter to make one pancake (you should be able to fit 4 pancakes in the skillet at a time). Cook until golden brown on both sides, 2 to 3 minutes per side. Repeat until all the batter is used.
6. Serve the pancakes with butter and maple syrup.

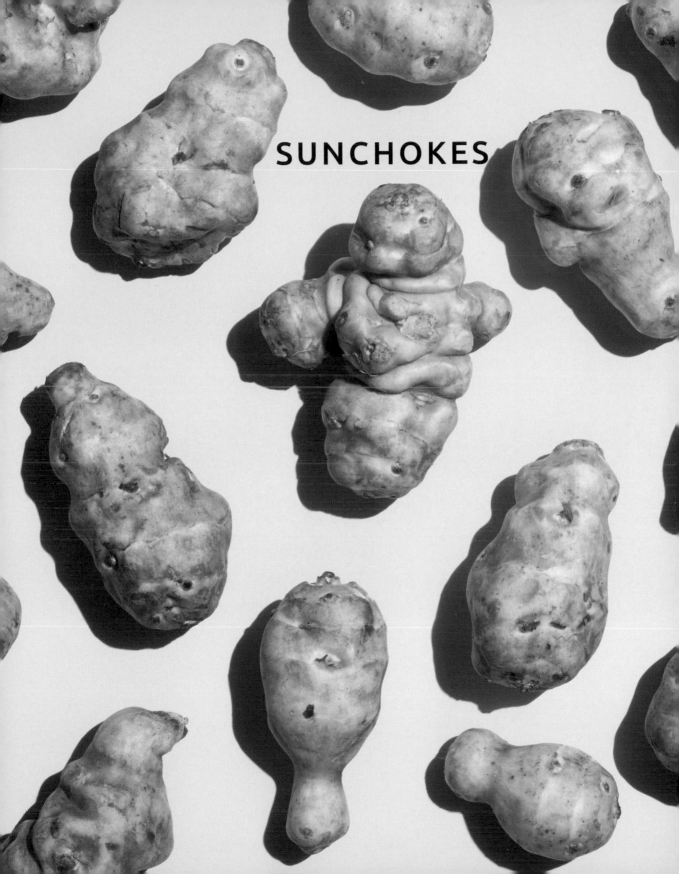

SUNCHOKES

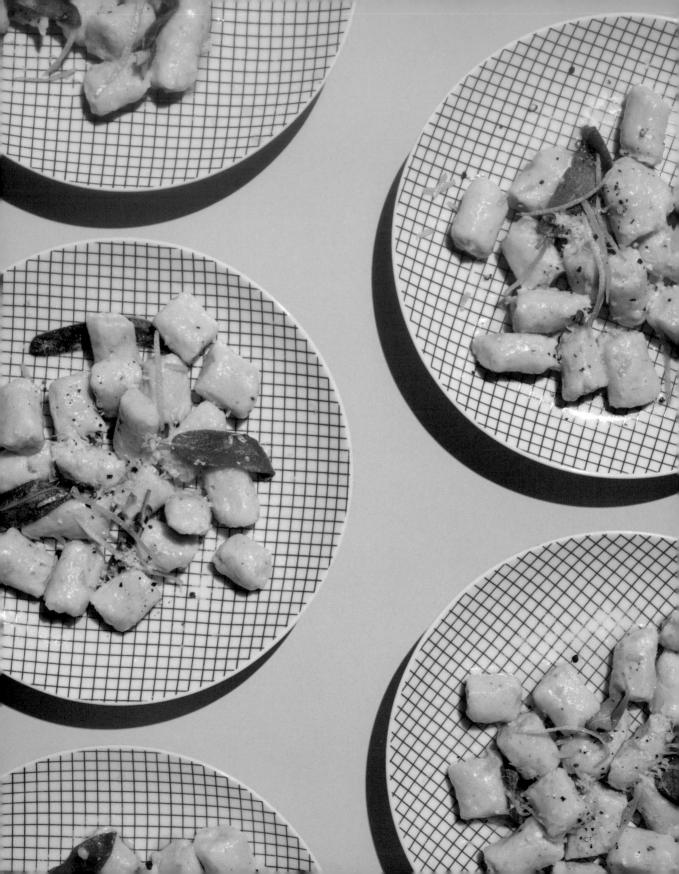

Sunchoke Gnocchi in a Lemon-Sage-Butter Sauce

Serves 4 to 6

Making gnocchi from scratch may seem intimidating, but it's really just pureeing some ingredients together and then squeezing out the contents into boiling water to cook for a few minutes. The sage-butter sauce is very impatient friendly, as well as totally delicious.

Kosher salt

2 pounds sunchokes, scrubbed clean and cut into 1-inch cubes

1 cup ricotta cheese

1 large egg

3 cups all-purpose flour

Freshly ground pepper

¼ pound (1 stick) unsalted butter

½ cup fresh sage leaves

1 lemon, zested and halved

½ cup grated Parmigiano-Reggiano cheese

1. Bring 2 pots of salted water to a boil (one for the sunchokes, the other for the gnocchi).
2. Add the sunchokes to one of the pots of boiling water and cook until tender, about 10 minutes. Drain and let cool, 5 to 10 minutes.
3. Transfer the sunchokes to a food processor and process until smooth. Add the ricotta, egg, flour, and 2 generous pinches of salt and pepper. Pulse a few times until evenly incorporated.
4. Remove the dough from the food processor and transfer into a large plastic storage bag. Push the dough down into one of the corners of the bag and cut 1 inch off the corner. Set aside.
5. In a large skillet, melt the butter over medium-high heat and cook until slightly browned, about 5 minutes. Add the sage and lemon zest and remove from the heat.
6. Pipe the sunchoke batter directly into the other pot of salted boiling water by squeezing the bag gently in one hand to force the dough out and cutting the dough into 1-inch segments just before they fall into the pot. Cook the gnocchi for about 4 minutes, until they float. Remove from the water using a slotted spoon or sieve and transfer to the butter sauce. Stir gently to coat the gnocchi in the sauce.
7. Serve the gnocchi with the grated Parmigiano and a squeeze of fresh lemon juice.

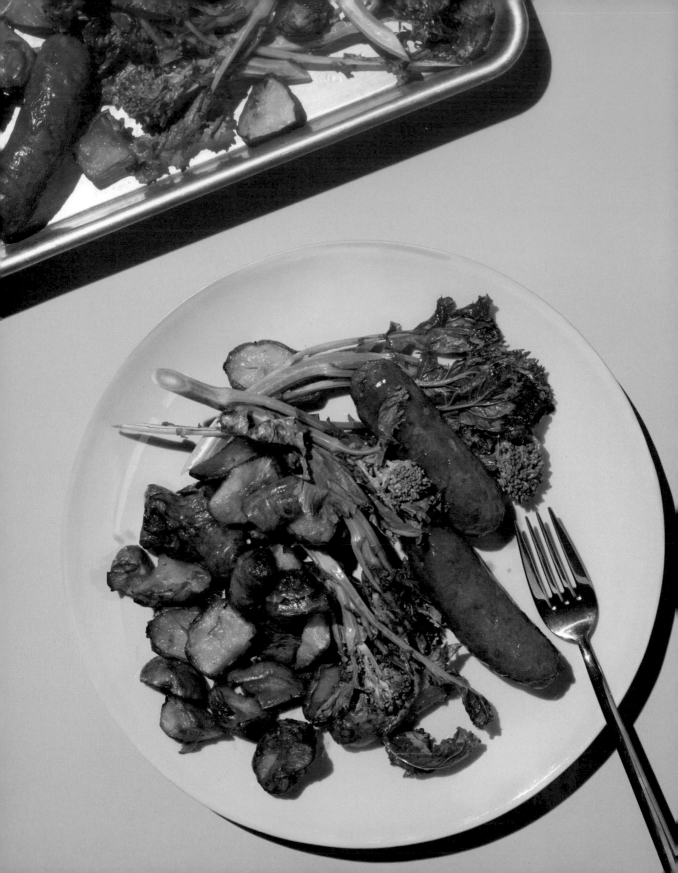

One-Sheet-Pan Meal:
Sunchokes, Rapini, Sausages

Serves 4 to 6

A one-sheet-pan meal is a recipe that can be baked on a single sheet pan (baking sheet with sides). It makes for the perfect impatient weeknight meal and keeps great as leftovers.

1 pound sunchokes, scrubbed
    clean and chopped into large
    bite-size pieces
2 tablespoons extra virgin olive oil
Kosher salt
4 links hot Italian sausage
1 bunch of broccoli rabe (rapini),
    ends trimmed
2 garlic cloves, thinly sliced
Freshly ground pepper
1 lemon, halved

1. Preheat the oven to 375°F.
2. Place the sunchokes on a 15 x 10-inch rimmed baking sheet and drizzle with 1 tablespoon of the olive oil and a generous pinch of salt. Transfer to the oven and set a timer for 10 minutes.
3. When the timer goes off, add the sausages to the pan and set the timer for another 10 minutes.
4. When the timer goes off, push the sunchokes and sausages to one side of the pan and add the broccoli rabe and garlic. Drizzle the remaining 1 tablespoon olive oil over the broccoli rabe and garlic, sprinkle with a pinch of salt, and bake for 10 more minutes, flipping the broccoli rabe over at the 5-minute mark so that it does not char.
5. Remove from the oven, transfer to plates, and top with some pepper. Squeeze a little fresh lemon juice over each serving. Enjoy!

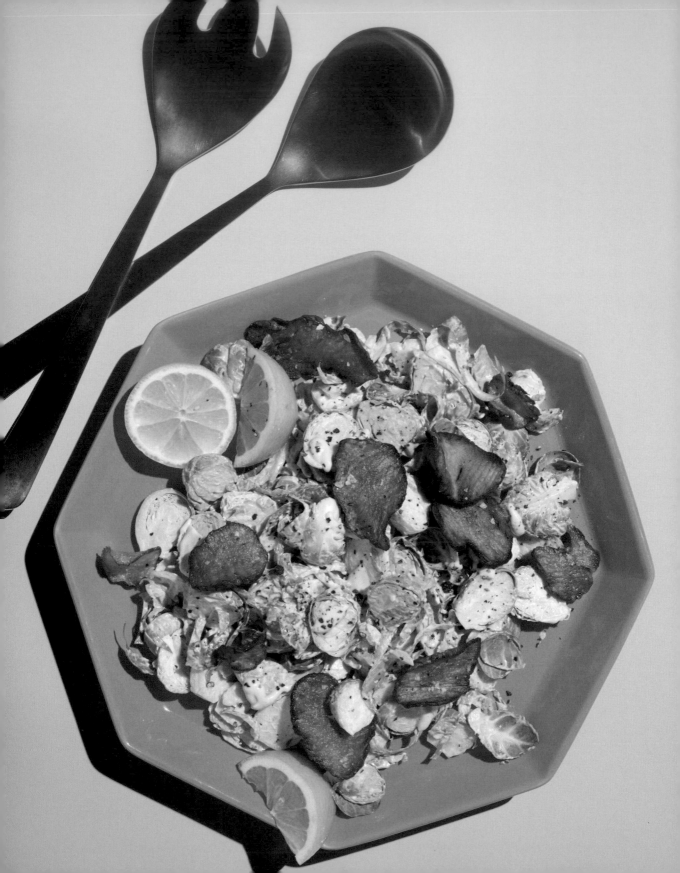

Winter Caesar Salad with Sunchoke Chips

Serves 4 to 6

For almost any other salad, you should wait to add the dressing until right before serving, otherwise the greens will get soggy and wilted. But this is one salad where you can mix in the dressing up to one hour ahead of time and store in the fridge until you are ready to serve.

1. Place the brussels sprouts in a large bowl. In a small bowl, whisk together the olive oil, yogurt, garlic, anchovy paste, lemon juice, and a pinch of salt and pepper. Add the dressing to the bowl of brussels sprouts and toss until the sprouts are evenly coated.
2. Make the sunchoke chips: In a skillet, heat the olive oil over medium-high heat. Add the sunchokes and cook until golden brown, about 5 minutes.
3. Garnish the salad with the sunchoke chips and serve.

2 pounds brussels sprouts, shredded on a mandoline or thinly sliced
4 tablespoons extra virgin olive oil
⅔ cup full-fat Greek yogurt
2 garlic cloves, minced
1 tablespoon anchovy paste
2 lemons, juiced
Kosher salt and freshly ground pepper

SUNCHOKE CHIPS
¼ cup extra virgin olive oil
½ pound sunchokes, scrubbed clean and sliced on a mandoline ¹⁄₁₆ inch thick

Sunchoke Soup

Serves 4 to 6

2 tablespoons extra virgin olive oil

2 garlic cloves, thinly sliced

2 tablespoons chopped fresh
   tarragon

½ cup white wine

3 to 4 small russet potatoes,
   peeled and cut into cubes

10 to 12 sunchokes, scrubbed
   clean and coarsely chopped

Kosher salt

4 cups low-sodium vegetable stock

The sunchokes help to make this vegan soup creamy, thick, and filling.

1. In a large pot, combine the olive oil, garlic, and 1 tablespoon of the tarragon. Cook over medium-high heat until the garlic is fragrant, 1 to 2 minutes.
2. Add the wine, potatoes, sunchokes, and 2 generous pinches of salt and stir together until the liquid has cooked off.
3. Add the vegetable stock and bring to a boil. Reduce the heat to a simmer, cover, and cook until the sunchokes and potatoes are soft, about 20 minutes.
4. Puree the soup with an immersion blender.
5. Serve garnished with the remaining 1 tablespoon of tarragon.

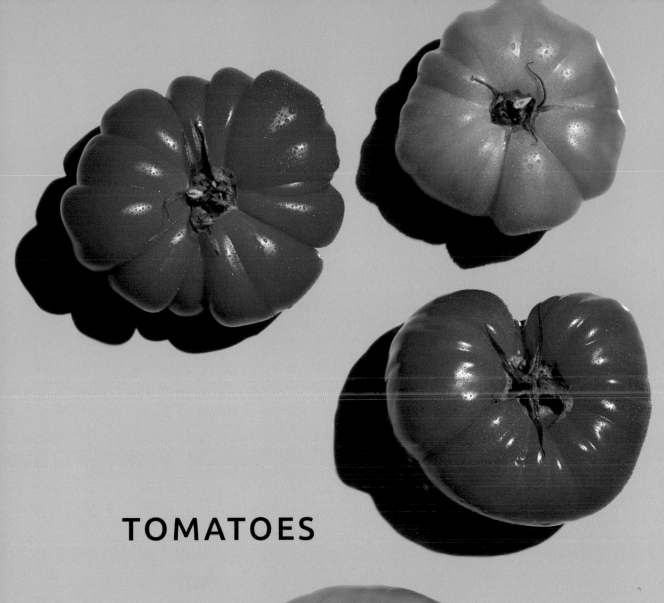

TOMATOES

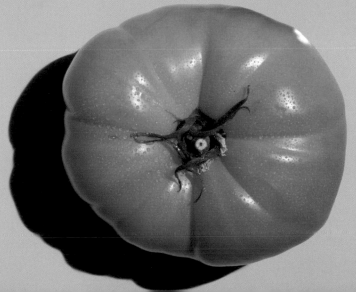

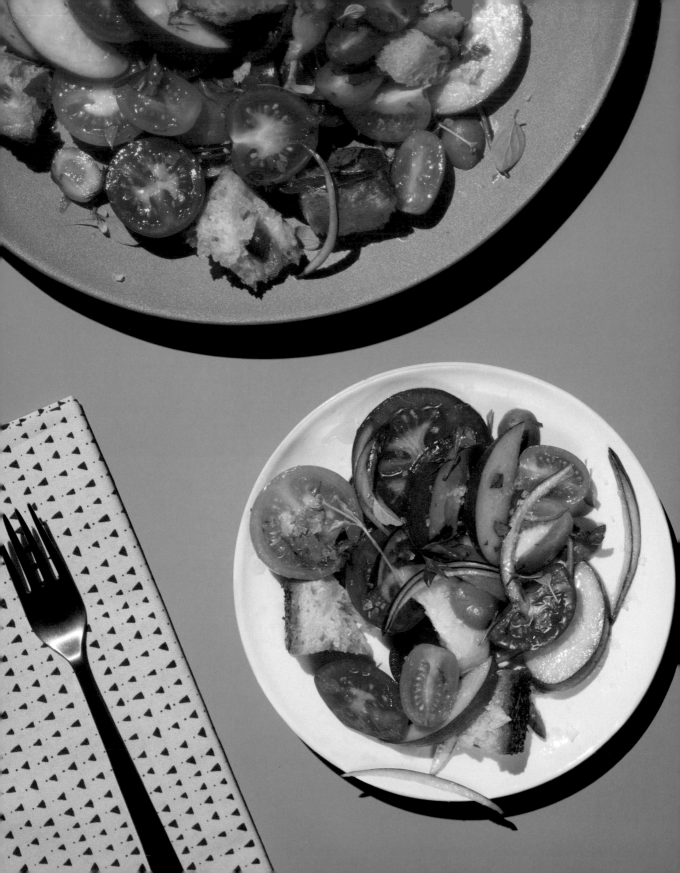

Claudia's Panzanella

Serves 4 to 6

Why serve a summer salad with bread on the side, when you can serve the bread in the salad? Panzanella is also a great way to make use of leftover bread or bread that is about to go stale.

1. Make the vinaigrette: In a small bowl, whisk together the olive oil, vinegar, salt, oregano, parsley, and dill.
2. Assemble the panzanella: Place the bread cubes, tomatoes, onion, peaches, and olives on a large platter. Add the vinaigrette and gently toss.

VINAIGRETTE

½ cup extra virgin olive oil

6 tablespoons red wine vinegar

1 tablespoon sea salt

2 tablespoons chopped fresh oregano

2 tablespoons chopped fresh flat leaf parsley

1 tablespoon chopped fresh dill

PANZANELLA

½ loaf crusty Italian bread, cut into cubes or torn into large bite-size pieces

2 cups mixed cherry tomatoes

6 vine tomatoes, each cut into 4 wedges

3 large mixed heirloom tomatoes, sliced thickly

1 small red onion, thinly sliced

4 peaches, sliced

½ cup Castelvetrano olives, pitted and sliced

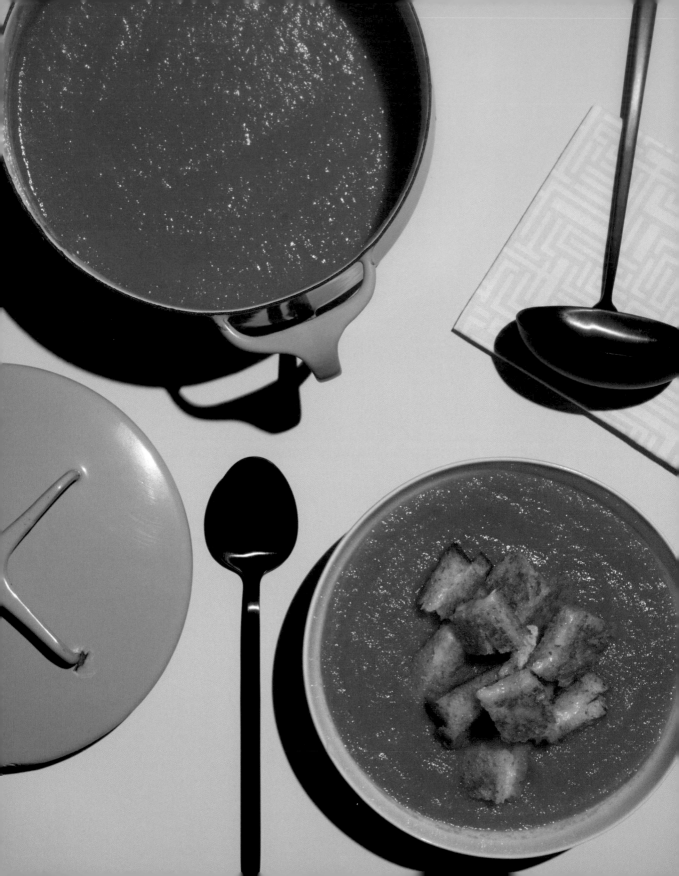

Tomato Soup with Grilled Cheese Croutons

Serves 4 to 6

The best bite is when the grilled cheese crouton gets absolutely soaked in the tomato soup—YUM.

1. In a large pot, combine the butter, olive oil, and basil and cook over medium heat until the basil is soft and fragrant, about 2 minutes. Remove and discard the basil.
2. Add the onion and garlic to the pot and cook, stirring frequently, until the onion is softened and translucent, about 5 minutes. Add a pinch of salt.
3. Add the fennel and carrots and cook, stirring occasionally, for 5 minutes.
4. Stir in the tomatoes and a pinch of salt and add 2 cups of water. Bring to a boil, then reduce to a simmer, cover, and cook for 20 minutes.
5. Meanwhile make the croutons: Spread one side of the bread with the butter. Transfer the bread, butter side down to a small or medium skillet and set over medium-high heat. Divide the cheddar between 2 of the slices, then top with the other slices of bread, this time butter-side up. Allow the sandwich to cook until the bread is golden and crispy and the cheese is completely melted, about 4 minutes per side. Cut into 1-inch cubes to make the croutons.
6. Once all the vegetables are tender, use an immersion blender or regular blender to puree the soup until very smooth. If the soup is too thick, add water ½ cup at a time until you reach the desired consistency. Season the soup with salt, pepper, and lemon juice to taste.
7. Pour the soup into bowls and divide the croutons evenly among the bowls.

1 tablespoon unsalted butter
1 tablespoon extra virgin olive oil
10 basil leaves
1 medium yellow onion, chopped
2 garlic cloves, minced
Kosher salt
1 bulb fennel (stalks, fronds, and outer leaves discarded), cut into ½-inch pieces
1 bunch of carrots, cut into ½-inch slices
8 Roma (plum) tomatoes, coarsely chopped
Freshly ground pepper
Fresh lemon juice

GRILLED CHEESE CROUTONS
4 slices sourdough bread
4 tablespoons (½ stick) unsalted butter, at room temperature
1 cup grated sharp cheddar cheese

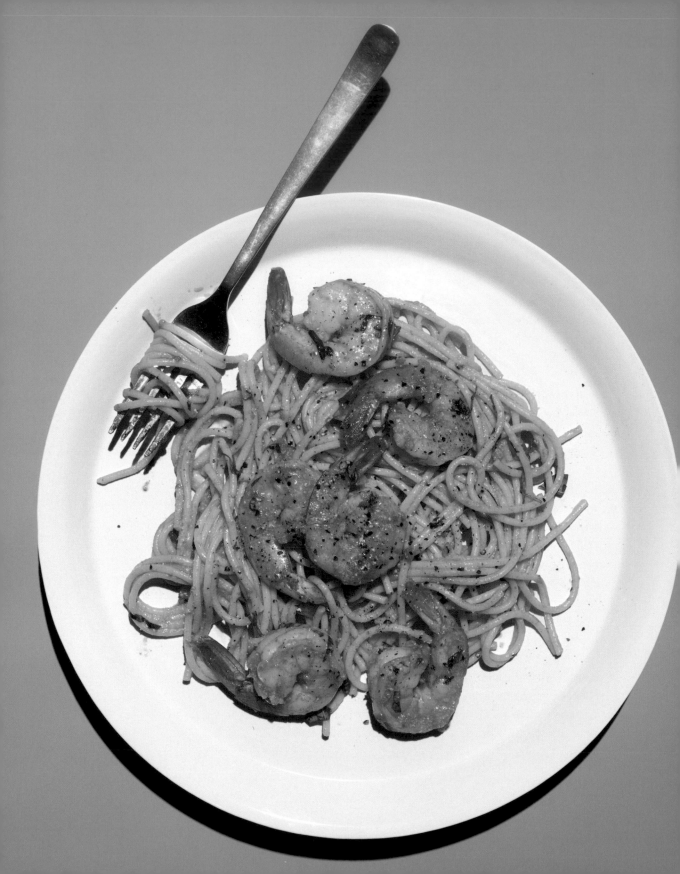

Spaghetti with Shrimp
in a Creamy Tomato-Saffron Sauce

Serves 4 to 6

I can feel the hot scorn of my Italian family for combining these flavors—they are very serious about what goes together and what absolutely does not. But damn it's delicious, and they're missing out.

Kosher salt

2 tablespoons extra virgin olive oil

1 medium yellow onion, chopped

2 garlic cloves, minced

½ teaspoon crumbled saffron
    threads

6 vine tomatoes, coarsely chopped

¼ teaspoon vanilla extract

1 pound spaghetti

1 pound shrimp, peeled and
    deveined

¼ cup full-fat Greek yogurt

½ cup packed fresh basil, minced

Freshly ground pepper

1. Bring a large pot of salted water to a boil.
2. In a large skillet, combine the olive oil, onion, garlic, and saffron and cook over medium heat until fragrant, about 3 minutes.
3. Add the tomatoes and vanilla and stir to combine. Reduce the heat to a simmer, cover, and set a timer for 20 minutes.
4. Add the spaghetti to the boiling water and cook according to the package directions.
5. When the timer goes off, add the shrimp to the sauce and cook, uncovered, until the shrimp turn pink, 3 to 4 minutes. Turn off the heat. Transfer the shrimp to a plate. Stir the yogurt into the tomato sauce until well combined.
6. Drain the spaghetti and transfer it to a large serving bowl. Top with the tomato sauce, some fresh basil, and pepper and toss to combine. Divide the spaghetti evenly among plates and top each plate with the shrimp.

An Impatient Bloody Mary

Makes 1 cocktail

¼ ounce fresh lemon juice
4 ounces Bloody Mary mix
1½ ounces vodka
Hot sauce
Cucumber slice, for garnish

For those mornings when you need the hair of the dog that bit you, plus some vitamins. (Lemon juice and cucumber count as vitamins, right?)

Pour the lemon juice, Bloody Mary mix, and vodka over ice, add hot sauce to taste, and garnish with a cucumber slice.

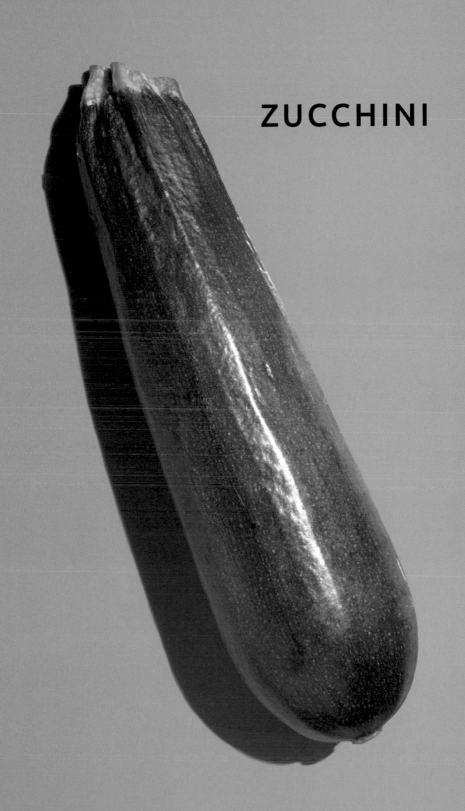

ZUCCHINI

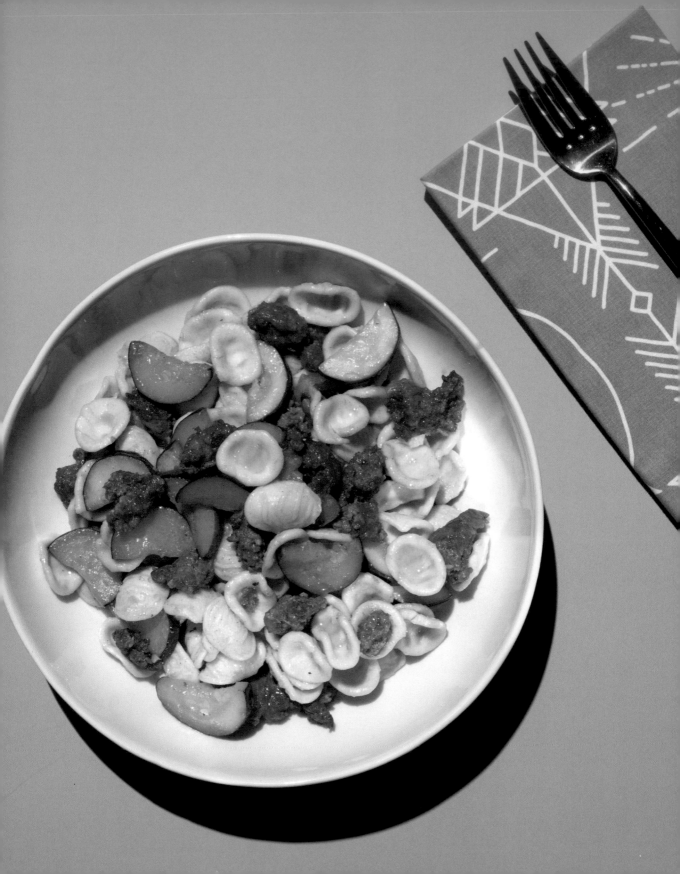

Five-Ingredient Zucchini Sausage Orecchiette

Serves 4 to 6

This recipe proves that you can make a filling and delicious meal with just five ingredients.

Kosher salt

4 tablespoons extra virgin olive oil

4 links hot Italian sausage, casings removed

4 zucchini, halved lengthwise, cut crosswise into ¼-inch-thick half-moons

1 pound orecchiette

Grated Parmigiano-Reggiano cheese, for serving

1. Bring a large pot of salted water to a boil.
2. In a large skillet, heat 2 tablespoons of the olive oil over medium-high heat. Add the sausage and cook, stirring constantly and breaking it up with a wooden spoon, about 4 minutes. Remove the sausage from the skillet and set aside.
3. Add 2 more tablespoons of the olive oil to the same skillet and heat over medium-high heat. Add the zucchini and cook until they are tender and slightly browned, about 10 minutes. Return the sausage to the skillet and remove from the heat.
4. Add the orecchiette to the boiling water and cook according to the package directions. Drain the orecchiette and add it to the skillet with the sausage and zucchini. Turn the heat to medium and gently toss to combine, about 2 minutes.
5. Serve in bowls with the Parmigiano.

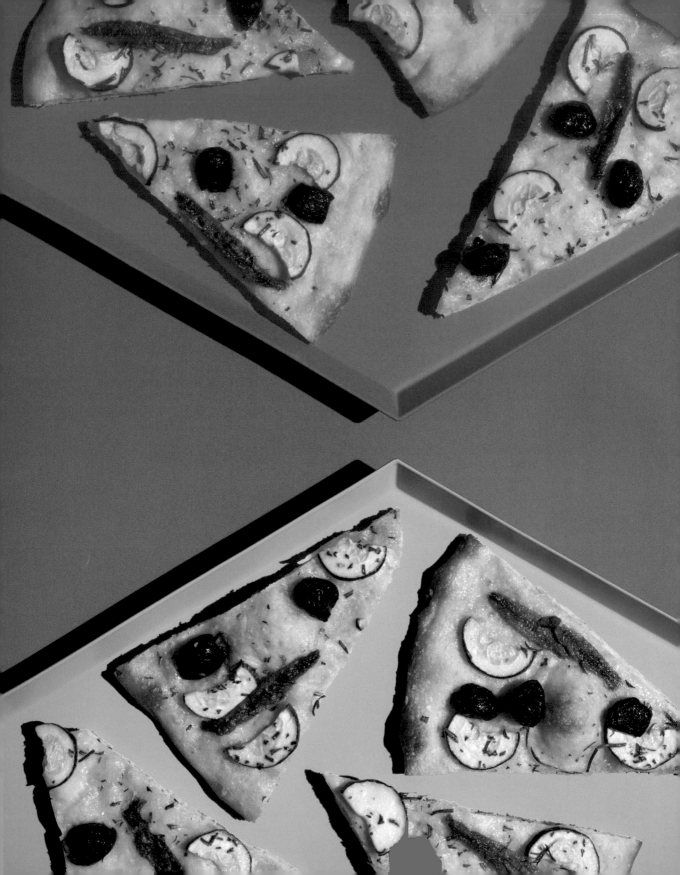

Zucchini Pizza with Black Olives, Anchovies, and Rosemary

Serves 4 to 6

This easy pizza is great as a lunch, a snack, or to bring on a picnic.

1. Preheat the oven to 400°F. Grease a 15 x 10-inch rimmed baking sheet with olive oil.
2. Press the pizza dough into the baking sheet to make a rectangle about ¼ inch thick (you will not take up the entire baking sheet). Brush the dough with olive oil and evenly scatter a pinch of salt over the dough.
3. In a medium bowl, toss the sliced zucchini with 2 tablespoons of olive oil and a pinch of salt.
4. Scatter the zucchini, olives, anchovy fillets, and rosemary over the dough. Bake until the crust is golden brown, about 20 minutes. Enjoy immediately or serve at room temperature or cold.

Extra virgin olive oil

1 pound store-bought fresh pizza dough

Kosher salt

1 zucchini, halved lengthwise, cut crosswise into ½-inch-thick half-moons

1 cup pitted black olives

1 (2-ounce) can anchovy fillets in olive oil

2 tablespoons chopped fresh rosemary

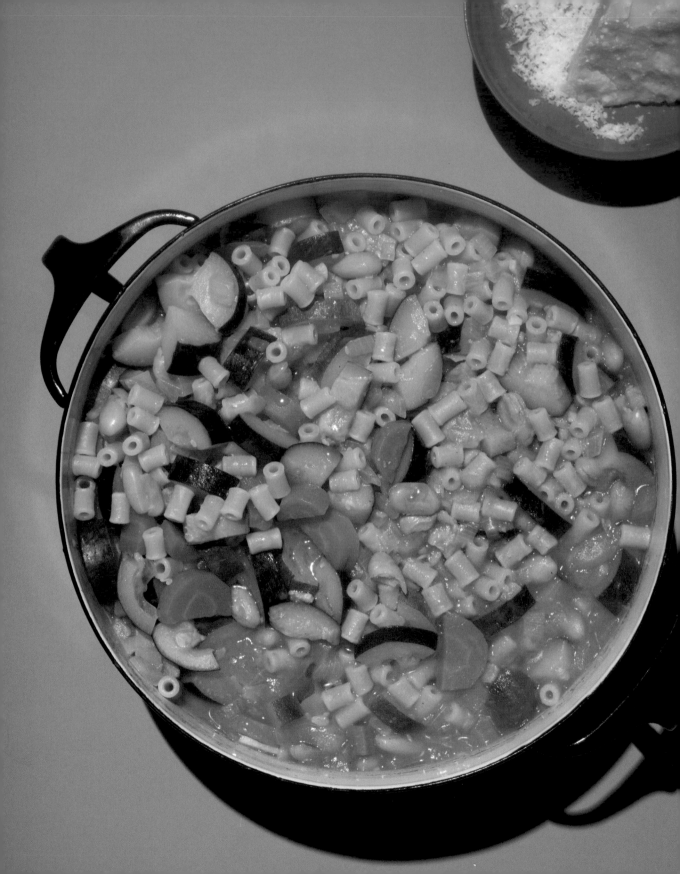

Zucchini Minestrone

Serves 4 to 6

Traditional minestrone has never been my favorite soup, but this version with zucchini makes it thicker and creamier, and turned me into a fan.

1. In a large pot, heat the olive oil over medium-high heat and add the onion, garlic, and carrots. Cook until fragrant and the onion is softened and translucent, about 3 minutes.
2. Add the zucchini, basil, vegetable stock, beans, tubetti, and 2 cups of water. Bring the broth to a boil, add 2 generous pinches of salt, then cover and cook until the tubetti are al dente, about 10 minutes.
3. Taste the soup, adding more salt and pepper, if needed.
4. Serve in bowls topped with a squeeze of fresh lemon juice and the Parmigiano.

2 tablespoons extra virgin olive oil
1 medium yellow onion, diced
2 garlic cloves, sliced
2 carrots, peeled, halved lengthwise, and cut crosswise
4 medium zucchini, halved lengthwise, cut crosswise into half-moons
1 cup chopped fresh basil
1 quart low-sodium vegetable stock
1 (15-ounce) can cannellini beans, drained and rinsed
8 ounces tubetti pasta
Kosher salt and freshly ground pepper
1 lemon, halved
1 cup grated Parmigiano-Reggiano cheese

Ginger and Orange Zucchini Bread

Serves 6 to 8

Butter, for greasing the pan

2 zucchini, grated on the large
     teardrops of a box grater

1 (16-ounce) box pound cake mix

Ingredients listed on the cake
     mix package for preparing the
     batter

2 oranges, zested and juiced

2 tablespoons finely grated fresh
     ginger (use a rasp-style zester)

1 tablespoon ground cinnamon

Whipped cream, for garnish
     (optional)

When making this recipe, it's very important to wring out the grated zucchini as much as possible—really put some elbow grease into it! If you don't do this properly, there is a risk that your zucchini bread will be a bust due to excess water.

1. Preheat the oven to 350°F. Butter a loaf pan and line with parchment paper, allowing excess parchment paper to come up above the long sides (this will allow for easy removal).
2. Wring out the grated zucchini in a clean kitchen towel and set aside.
3. Make the pound cake mix according to the package directions, replacing the liquid called for with the orange juice. If there is not enough orange juice, add water or milk to meet the liquid requirement. Add the orange zest, ginger, cinnamon, and zucchini to the batter and mix.
4. Scrape the batter into the prepared pan and bake until a toothpick comes out clean, about 35 minutes.
5. Let the zucchini bread cool before serving. This would be excellent with some whipped cream!

CHICKEN, MEAT, FISH

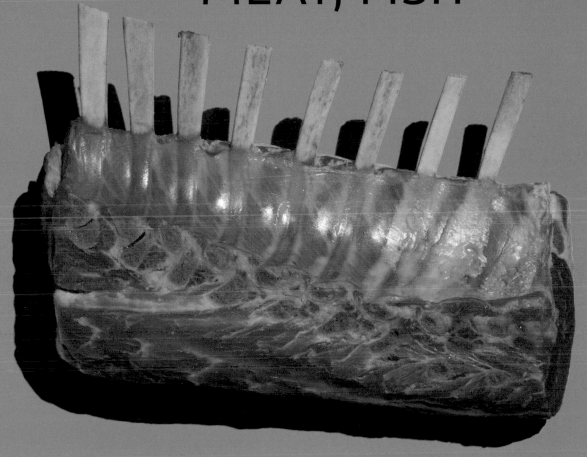

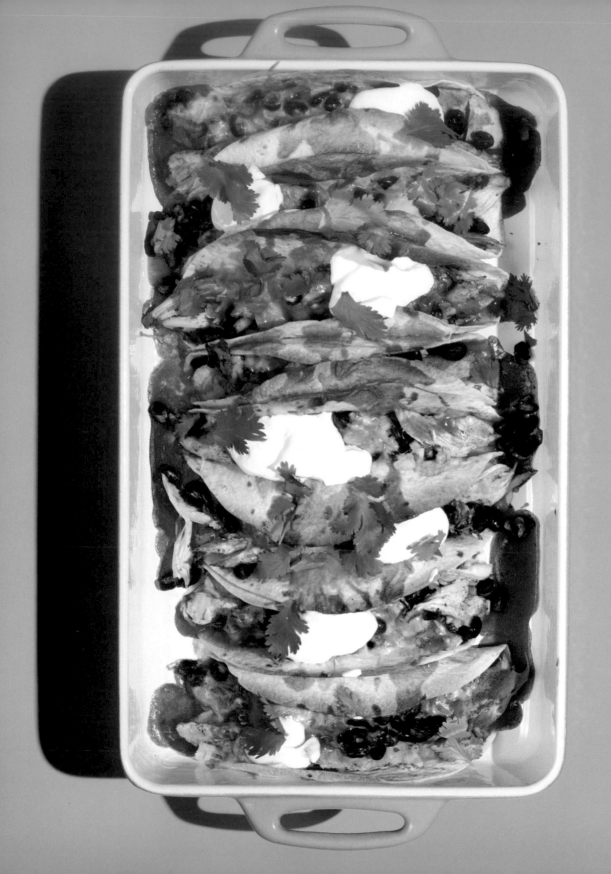

Thury's Impatient Baked Enchiladas

Serves 6 to 8

My stepmother is an Icelandic wonder woman who does a million things and also somehow has found the time to qualify and compete in two Ironman championships at Kona. This is a recipe she makes for her three kids when time (and patience) is tight.

1. Preheat the oven to 350°F. Lightly grease the inside of a shallow rectangular (1-quart) casserole dish.
2. Fold the tortillas in half and stand them, side by side, with the curved side down in the casserole dish. (Each should look like a "U" or a taco shell.)
3. Spoon the chicken, beans, a pinch of salt, some onion, and cilantro evenly into each tortilla.
4. Pour the enchilada sauce evenly over everything and sprinkle evenly with the cheese. The tortillas will still be sticking out the top.
5. Bake until the tortillas get a little crisp at the edges, about 20 minutes.
6. Use a spatula to transfer the enchiladas to a plate. Garnish with the reserved cilantro and a dollop of sour cream. Enjoy immediately!

Olive oil, for greasing the pan
8 (8-inch) flour tortillas
1 store-bought rotisserie chicken, meat torn into bite-size pieces
1 (15.5-ounce) can black beans or pinto beans, drained and rinsed
Kosher salt
1 small yellow onion, finely chopped
1 cup fresh cilantro, chopped (reserve some for garnish)
1 (10-ounce) can red or green enchilada sauce
1 (6-ounce) package shredded Mexican cheese blend
Sour cream

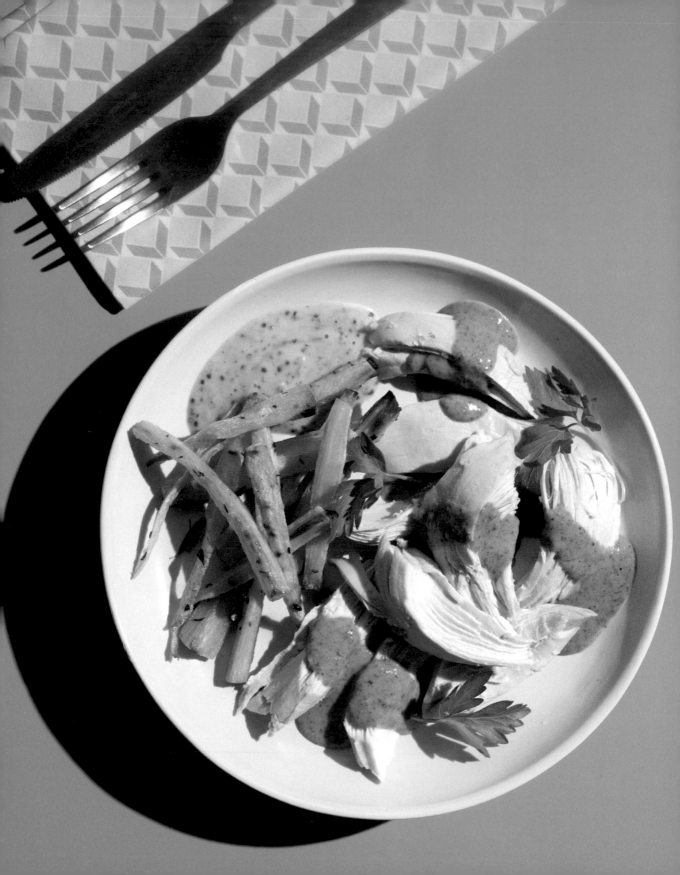

Camilla's Bollito with Salsa Verde

Serves 2 to 4

I know that the cooking time on this is on the longer side, but I included it in this book because it's a recipe that pays dividends: It's great just out of the pot, or as leftovers, in the form of moist chicken shredded onto a salad, or sliced into a sandwich. You can also mix the salsa verde with mayo to make a nice spread for a sandwich. The recipe comes from my mom's childhood friend, Camilla Toniolo.

1. Prepare the chicken: In a large stockpot, combine the chicken, onion, carrots, celery, leek, parsley stems, and 2 generous pinches of salt. Add enough cold water to cover all the ingredients. Cover the pot and bring to a boil over high heat. Reduce the heat to a gentle simmer, cover, and cook for at least 1½ hours. Skim off the scum with a spoon every 20 minutes.

2. While the chicken is cooking, make the salsa verde: Scoop out the center of the bread to get 1 cup (discard the crust). Soak the bread in the vinegar plus ¼ cup water for 10 minutes. Wring the liquid out of the bread with your hands.

3. In a food processor, combine the bread, parsley, capers, egg, anchovy paste, garlic, salt, and pepper and process to break up and combine the ingredients.

4. Gradually add the olive oil through the feed tube while pulsing until the salsa verde comes together. Refrigerate until ready to use.

5. When the chicken is cooked, remove it from the pot and cut it into serving pieces. Arrange them on a platter and top with the salsa verde.

6. You will have a potful of chicken broth. Strain it (discard the vegetables) and freeze for future use.

CHICKEN

1 whole chicken (about 4 pounds)
1 medium yellow onion, skin-on, halved
2 carrots, unpeeled
2 celery stalks, halved
1 leek, cleaned and halved lengthwise
A handful of fresh flat leaf parsley stems
Kosher salt

SALSA VERDE

1 large bread roll
¼ cup white wine vinegar
1 cup packed fresh flat leaf parsley leaves
¼ cup capers
1 large egg, hard-boiled
1 teaspoon anchovy paste
1 garlic clove, peeled
½ teaspoon kosher salt
½ teaspoon freshly ground pepper
½ cup extra virgin olive oil

Chou's Vinegar Chicken

Serves 4 to 6

8 to 10 chicken drumsticks

Kosher salt

¼ bottle dry white wine

1 heaping tablespoon tomato
    paste

1 tablespoon Dijon mustard

Freshly ground pepper

1 tablespoon unsalted butter

1 tablespoon sunflower oil

6 garlic cloves, peeled

½ cup balsamic vinegar

2 tablespoons heavy cream
    (optional)

This recipe was one of the first "grown-up" recipes I learned. It was taught to me by a babysitter I had for many years named Geraldine, whom I affectionately called Chou. She taught me this when I was about twelve years old and, to this day, it's one of my favorite meals. Even if you don't use the heavy cream, the sauce is incredibly rich.

1. Remove the drumsticks from the fridge to bring to room temperature. Pat them with paper towels to remove excess moisture, sprinkle evenly with salt, and set aside. Place some paper towels on a clean plate and set aside.

2. Meanwhile, in a bowl, combine the wine, tomato paste, mustard, and a pinch of salt and pepper and whisk to combine. Set aside.

3. In a large skillet, heat the butter and oil over medium-high heat. You want the butter to be melted and bubbling, but not browning.

4. When the butter and oil are hot, sear the drumsticks, turning every few minutes, until the skin is golden brown and crispy, 8 to 10 minutes. Add the garlic toward the end of the browning. (You may have to cook the drumsticks in batches.) Move the browned drumsticks to the plate with the paper towels.

5. Pour the vinegar into the skillet and deglaze the pan (aka scrape the bottom of the pan with a wooden spoon while the vinegar cooks off to get all the yummy, crispy pieces off the bottom of the pan). When the vinegar is reduced, return the drumsticks to the pan.

6. Pour the wine mixture over the drumsticks and reduce the

heat to medium-low. Cook, uncovered, for about 30 minutes, turning the drumsticks every 10 minutes or so to ensure they cook evenly.

7. If you are using the heavy cream, add it about 2 minutes before you remove the drumsticks from the heat.

8. Season with salt and pepper to taste and transfer the drumsticks to a serving platter. Pour all the yummy sauce and garlic cloves over the drumsticks. Enjoy.

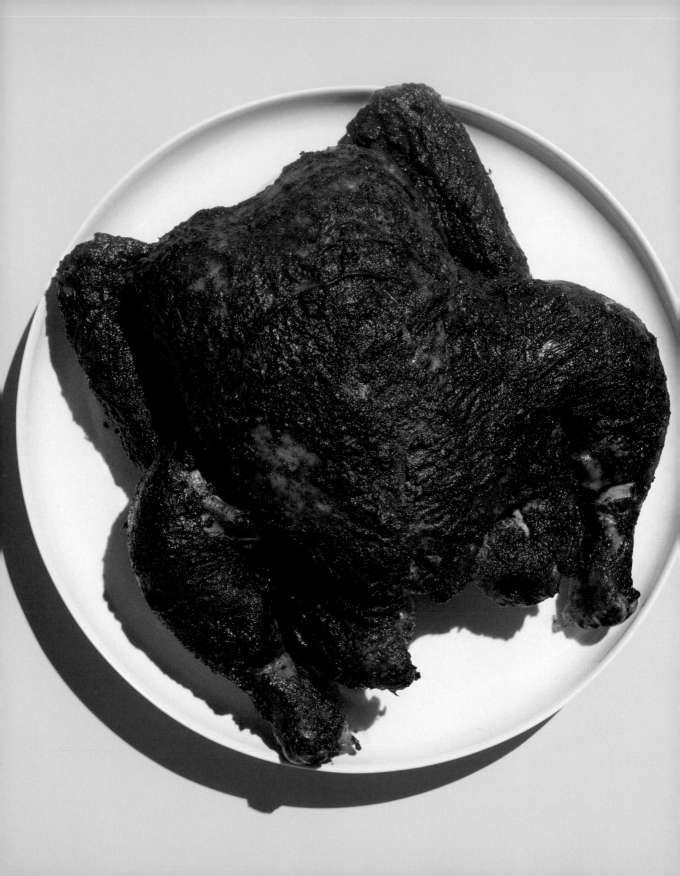

Useless Spice Split Roast Chicken

Serves 2 to 4

A cookbook directed me to purchase five-spice powder, assuring me I would absolutely love this spice and use it all the time. Then it sat and gathered dust in my pantry for four-plus years. Every time I opened it to smell it, my mind would flash question marks—I don't think the cookbook itself had any recipes using this spice! If you fell into a similar trap and have this spice floating around your kitchen, this chicken recipe is for you.

3 tablespoons extra virgin olive oil
2 tablespoons soy sauce
1 teaspoon Sriracha sauce
½ teaspoon grated fresh ginger
1 garlic clove, grated
½ lime, juiced
2 tablespoons five-spice powder
¼ teaspoon cayenne pepper
1 whole chicken (about 4 pounds),
    spatchcocked (ask your
    butcher to do this)
Kosher salt

1. Preheat the oven to 450°F. Grease a 12-inch ovenproof pan or cast iron skillet with 1 tablespoon of the olive oil.
2. Make a wet rub by combining the remaining 2 tablespoons of olive oil, the soy sauce, Sriracha, ginger, garlic, lime juice, five-spice powder, and cayenne.
3. Pat the chicken down with paper towels until it is very dry. The drier the skin the crispier it will become in the oven!
4. Lay the chicken in the skillet, breast-side up. Season generously with salt and massage the wet rub all over the chicken to coat evenly. Tuck the wings under the body so they don't burn.
5. Roast for 45 minutes, or until an instant-read thermometer inserted into the thickest part of the thigh registers 165°F. (Don't let the thermometer touch the bone, or you might get an inaccurate reading.) When the chicken is done roasting, allow it to rest for 10 minutes—this will make the chicken even juicier!
6. Serve the chicken with the pan juices on the side.

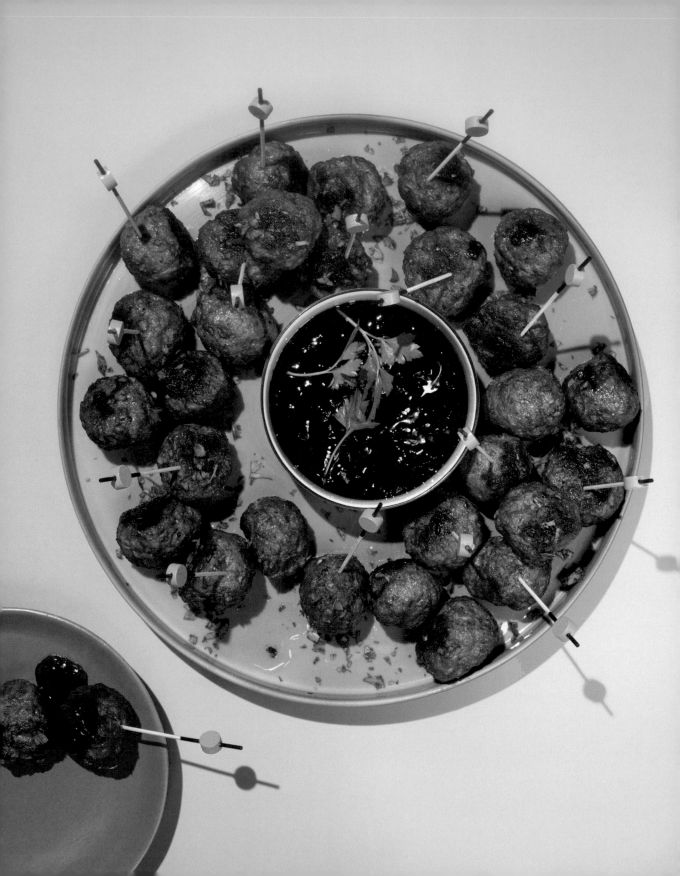

Swedish Meatballs

Serves 4 to 6

This recipe comes from a dear family friend, Paavo Turtianinen. He has cooked these meatballs for three generations of my mom's side of the family, and they are a hit every time.

1 pound lean ground beef
½ pound ground pork
½ cup unseasoned dried bread crumbs
1 small yellow onion, grated on the large teardrops of a box grater
¼ cup heavy cream
5 tablespoons chopped fresh flat leaf parsley
1 teaspoon kosher salt
¼ teaspoon freshly ground pepper
¼ teaspoon ground allspice
Red currant jelly, for serving (optional)

1. Preheat the oven to 400°F. Line a 15 x 10-inch baking sheet with parchment paper.
2. In large bowl, combine the ground beef, ground pork, bread crumbs, onion, cream, 3 tablespoons of the parsley, the salt, pepper, and allspice.
3. Shape into 1½-inch balls and place on the baking sheet, evenly spaced. (The mixture should yield about 24 meatballs.)
4. Bake for 20 minutes, or until an instant-read thermometer inserted into the center of a meatball registers 160°F.
5. Garnish with the remaining parsley and serve with red currant jelly, if desired.

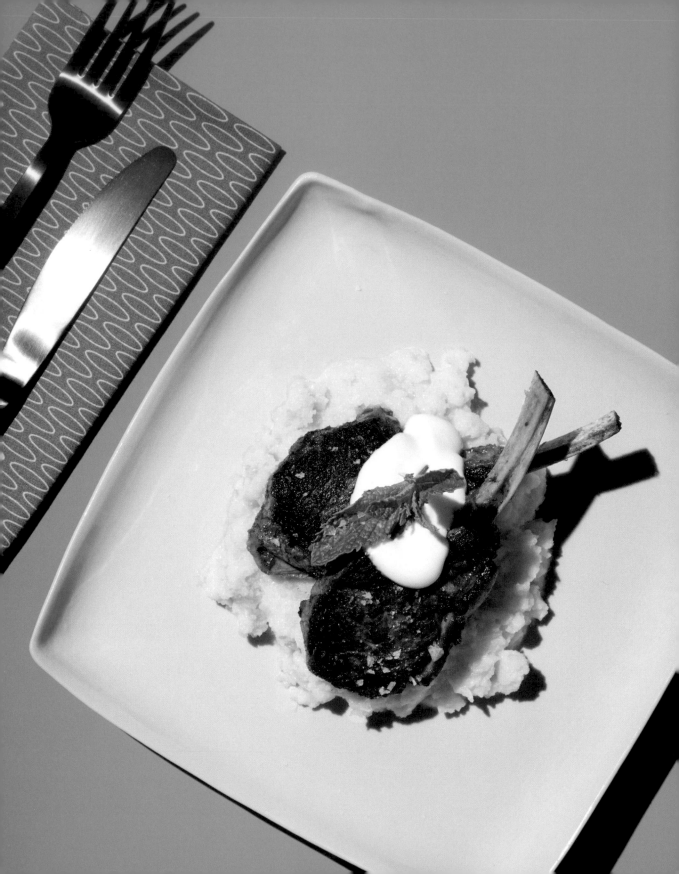

Harissa Lamb Chops with Mashed Cauliflower

Serves 4

The great thing about lamb chops is that they take just a few minutes to cook, so sear them as your last step! We tested these chops after being marinated for a few minutes and also after a few hours. The longer the marination time, the stronger the flavors, obviously, but both options were flavorful and delicious.

1. Prepare the chops: In a small bowl, combine the olive oil, harissa, lemon zest, and a small pinch of salt. Place the chops in a zip-seal plastic bag or in a large bowl and pour the marinade over the chops, rubbing to coat evenly. Set the chops aside at room temperature to marinate. If you are not eating the chops until much later, marinate them in the fridge.

2. Meanwhile, make the cauliflower: Bring a large pot of water to a boil. Add the cauliflower and cook until soft, 8 to 9 minutes. Drain the cauliflower and return it to the pot. Add the stock and butter and puree until smooth with an immersion blender or food processor. You want it to be the consistency of mashed potatoes. Set aside.

3. To finish: In a large skillet, heat the vegetable oil over high heat. Working in two batches if necessary, add the chops, searing on both sides, 1 to 2 minutes per side. Make sure not to crowd the chops.

4. On each of 4 dinner plates, serve ½ cup of the cauliflower mash with 2 chops on top. Top with a dollop of yogurt and a sprinkle of the fresh mint. Serve immediately.

HARISSA LAMB CHOPS
½ cup extra virgin olive oil
¼ cup harissa
Zest of 1 lemon
Kosher salt
8 lamb chops
2 tablespoons vegetable oil

CAULIFLOWER MASH
1 head of cauliflower, broken into florets and chopped
¼ cup low-sodium vegetable or chicken stock
2 tablespoons unsalted butter

FOR SERVING
½ cup full-fat Greek yogurt
Fresh mint leaves, chopped

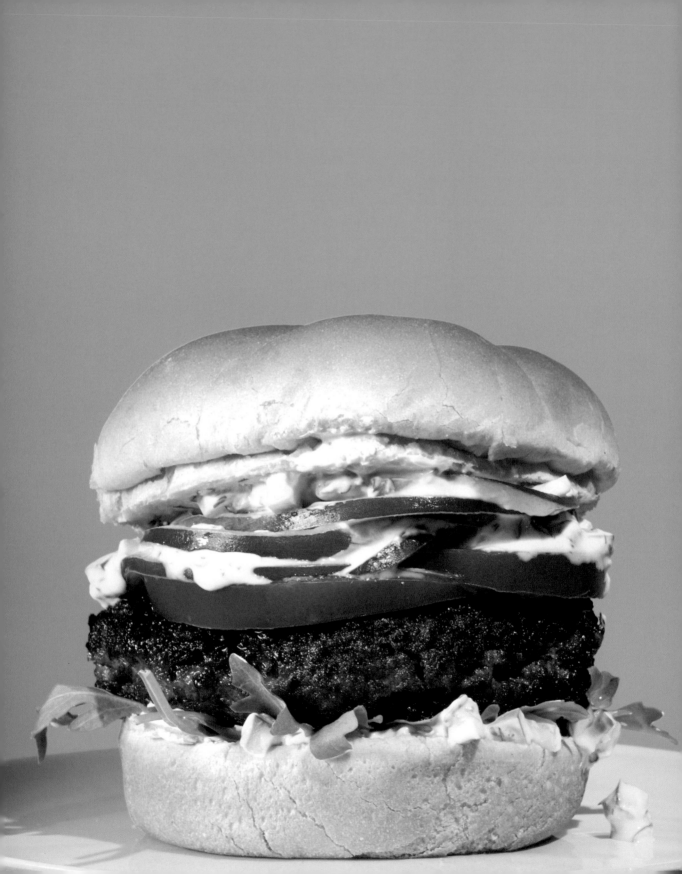

Greek Lamb Burger with Pickled Red Onion and Tzatziki

Serves 4

If you're feeling impatient or pressed for time, you can buy tzatziki at many grocery stores and cut that step out entirely. Making pickled onions requires nothing more than slicing an onion and letting it marinate and the burgers come together quickly and easily.

1. Make the tzatziki: Place the cucumber in a medium bowl. Add the yogurt, dill, lemon juice, and garlic and stir to combine. Set aside.
2. Make the pickled onions: In a bowl, combine the vinegar and sugar. Add the onion and allow to pickle while you make the burgers.
3. Prepare the burgers: In a large bowl, combine the lamb, onion, lemon zest, oregano, rosemary, and generous pinch of salt and pepper. Using your hands, mix all the ingredients together and form 4 patties.
4. In a large skillet, heat the olive oil over medium-high heat. Add the lamb patties and sear for 3 minutes per side. Don't pester them, just let them cook undisturbed.
5. To serve, place some tzatziki on the bottom half of each burger bun, then add arugula, a lamb burger, and a tomato slice. Pinch the red onion out of the pickling liquid and place on top of the tomato. Top with a dollop of tzatziki. Close your burger and enjoy.

TZATZIKI
½ small English (seedless) cucumber, finely chopped
½ cup full-fat Greek yogurt
2 tablespoons chopped fresh dill
½ lemon, juiced
1 small garlic clove, grated on a rasp-style zester

PICKLED ONION
½ cup distilled white vinegar
2 tablespoons sugar
½ large red onion, thinly sliced

LAMB BURGERS
1 pound ground lamb
½ small red onion, finely chopped
Zest of 1 lemon
2 tablespoons chopped fresh oregano
2 tablespoons chopped fresh rosemary
Kosher salt and freshly ground pepper
2 tablespoons extra virgin olive oil

FOR SERVING
1 cup arugula
4 burger buns
1 tomato, sliced

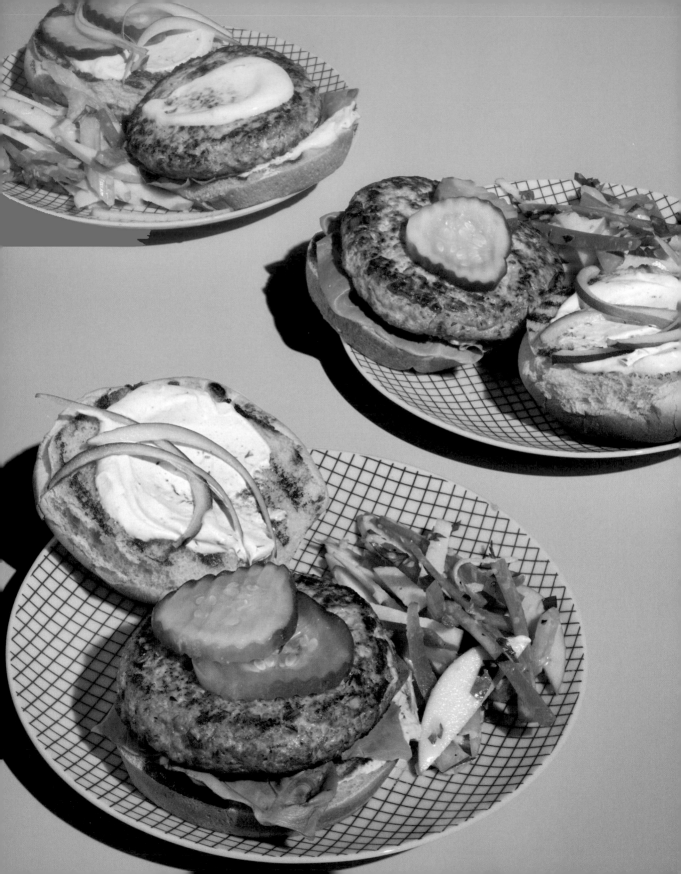

Claudia's Salmon Burgers

Serves 4

If your experience of salmon burgers to date has been out of the frozen foods aisle, this easy recipe will show you what salmon burgers really can be and what they are meant to be. They're impatient foodie–friendly, impressive, delicious, and healthy—a win all around. My little brother and sister—not normally fish fans—gobbled these up and asked for seconds.

1. Cut the salmon fillet into 1½-inch-wide chunks. Place in a food processor. Add the scallions, dill pickles, dill, mustard, 2 generous pinches of salt, and a few turns of pepper. Pulse 10 times, until the mixture is coarse. Add the yogurt and pulse until just combined.
2. Transfer the mixture to a medium bowl and divide into 4 equal balls.
3. In a 12-inch skillet, heat the olive oil over medium-high heat. Place all 4 salmon balls in the skillet and press down lightly with a spatula to form patties. Cook until golden and crispy on both sides, about 8 minutes total (see Note).
4. Meanwhile, make the sauce: In a small bowl, combine the yogurt, Sriracha, pickle juice, and dill. Set aside.
5. For serving, toast the burger buns. Smear a generous dollop of Claudia's secret sauce on both sides of the bun. Place a lettuce leaf on the bottom bun, top with a salmon patty, 2 pickle rounds per sandwich, and some red onion. Enjoy immediately!

SALMON PATTIES

1 pound salmon fillet, skinned
2 scallions, sliced
6 dill pickle slices (rounds)
2 heaping tablespoons chopped fresh dill
1 teaspoon Dijon mustard
Kosher salt and freshly ground pepper
¼ cup full-fat Greek yogurt
2 tablespoons extra virgin olive oil

CLAUDIA'S SECRET SAUCE

½ cup full-fat Greek yogurt
1 tablespoon Sriracha sauce
2 tablespoons pickle juice
1 teaspoon chopped fresh dill

FOR SERVING

4 burger buns
4 butter lettuce leaves
8 dill pickle slices (rounds)
¼ red onion, thinly sliced

NOTE: Resist the temptation to poke and pester the burgers as they are cooking—just set a timer and leave them alone.

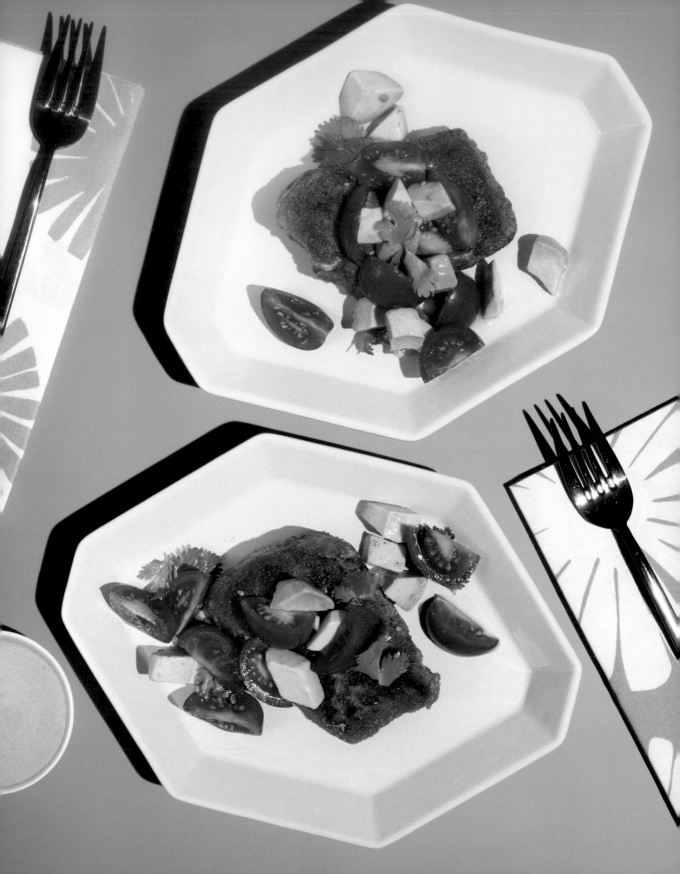

Almond-Crusted Cod on a Tomato and Avocado Salad

Serves 4

This recipe is longer on the ingredient side, but don't let that scare you! The salad shouldn't take more than 10 minutes to prepare, and the fish prep takes 10 to 15 minutes as well. Many of these ingredients are quickly combined to make the spiced-flour coating for the fish, so minimal fuss (and minimal dishes). When cooking fish in a skillet, it's important to remember not to pester it—don't poke it with a spatula or move the pan around. You risk breaking up the fish into smaller pieces and not having it cook evenly.

1. Make the salad: In a large bowl, combine the olive oil, tomatoes, avocado, lemon juice, cilantro, and a generous pinch of salt and pepper. Stir gently to combine. Set aside.
2. Make the sauce: Stir together the Sriracha, mayonnaise, and lemon juice. Set aside.
3. Prepare the cod: In a small bowl, combine the almond flour, cumin, curry powder, and 2 generous pinches of salt and stir to mix. In a separate small bowl, whisk the egg and milk to combine.
4. Coat the fish first in the egg mixture and then roll in the almond flour mixture to coat evenly.
5. In a large skillet, heat the vegetable oil over medium-high heat. Add the fish and cook until the breading is golden and crispy, about 3 minutes per side. Remember to resist the temptation to move the fish around too much—just let it cook!
6. To plate, place a piece of fish atop some of the tomato and avocado salad and drizzle the sauce on the fish. Serve immediately.

SALAD

2 tablespoons extra virgin olive oil
12 Campari tomatoes, quartered
2 avocados, cut into cubes
1 lemon, juiced
½ cup chopped fresh cilantro
Kosher salt and freshly ground
    pepper

SAUCE

¼ cup Sriracha sauce
½ cup mayonnaise
1 lemon, juiced

ALMOND-CRUSTED COD

1 cup almond flour
1 tablespoon ground cumin
1 tablespoon curry powder
Kosher salt
1 large egg
¼ cup whole milk or water
1 pound cod, cut into 4 pieces
    (or black sea bass, halibut, or
    whatever flaky white fish is in
    season)
2 tablespoons vegetable oil

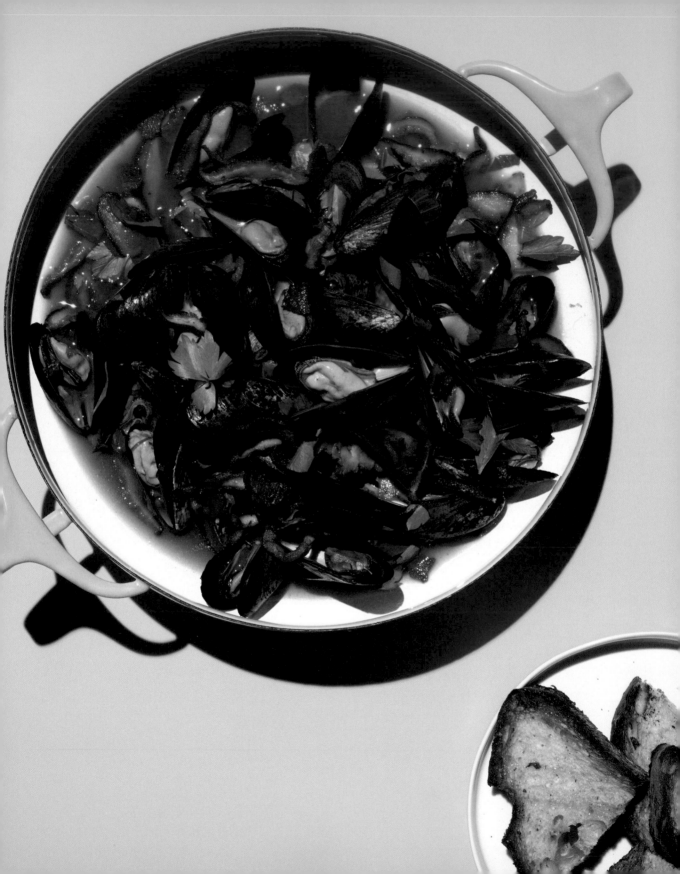

Impatient Mussels in Mushroom Broth

Serves 4 to 6

Garlic bread would be an excellent addition here. An impatient version of garlic bread is minimal fuss: Simply toast some thick sliced bread and rub a garlic clove all over it, top with butter, and keep the bread warm in a 200°F oven until the soup is ready.

¼ cup dried porcini mushrooms
2 slices bacon, chopped
½ cup sliced shiitake mushroom caps
1 small white onion, chopped
4 sprigs of fresh sage, leaves picked and chopped
Kosher salt and freshly ground pepper
½ cup white wine
2 pounds mussels, rinsed, beards pulled, open shells discarded
¼ cup chopped fresh flat leaf parsley

1. In a small saucepan, bring 1 cup of water to a boil. Add the porcinis, remove from the heat, and set aside to soften.
2. In a large pot, over medium-low heat, cook the bacon until it starts to crisp, about 10 minutes. Add the shiitakes and allow them to brown, about 4 minutes. Add the onion, sage, and a generous pinch of salt and pepper. Cook until the onion softens, about 5 minutes. Add the wine to deglaze the pot.
3. Meanwhile, fish the porcinis out of the soaking water. Strain the soaking water through a paper towel into the pot. Chop the porcini mushrooms and add them to the pot as well.
4. Bring the liquid to a boil, then add the mussels. Give one quick stir and cover. Cook until the mussels open wide, 3 to 5 minutes. Discard any mussels that do not open.
5. Serve the mussels in bowls with some broth and garnish with the parsley.

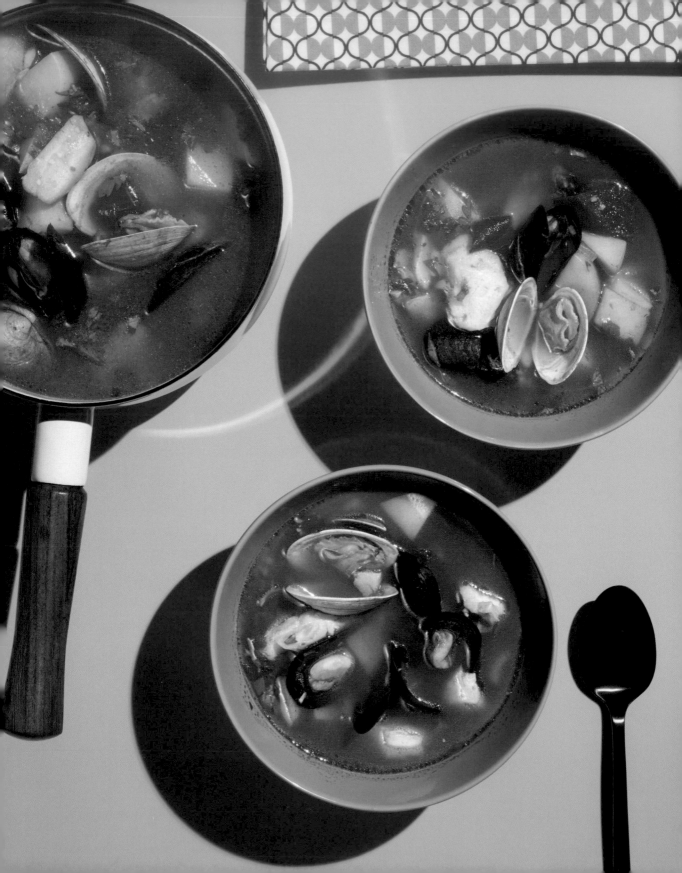

Impatient Fish Stew

Serves 4 to 6

The first time I had bouillabaisse was with my grandparents at a restaurant in NYC when I was in my early twenties. I went home and immediately looked up how to make it. Two hours of cooking time?! HA! No way, José. Years later, we figured out a (very) impatient version.

1. Run the mussels and clams under running water, scrubbing with a brush or coarse sponge if they're dirty and removing any beards from the mussels with your fingers. Discard any mussels or clams that stay open when you tap them, or any with broken shells.

2. In a large pot, heat the 2 tablespoons olive oil over medium heat. Add the shallots and sauté until fragrant and softened, 2 to 3 minutes.

3. Add the potatoes, tomatoes, saffron, and 2 generous pinches of salt and stir to combine. Pour in the fish stock, increase the heat to high, cover, and bring to a boil.

4. Meanwhile, toast the country bread, then rub the cut garlic over them, adding a drizzle of olive oil. Set aside.

5. When the broth is boiling, add the mussels, clams, and cod. Reduce the heat to a simmer, cover, and cook until the mussels and clams open, about 5 minutes.

6. Serve immediately with the garlic bread.

½ pound mussels
½ pound manila clams
2 tablespoons extra virgin olive oil, plus more for drizzling
2 shallots, finely chopped
6 baby potatoes, quartered
2 vine tomatoes, coarsely chopped
½ teaspoon saffron threads
Kosher salt
6 cups low-sodium fish stock
6 to 8 slices country bread
3 garlic cloves, halved
2 pounds cod fillets, cut into bite-size chunks

Impatient Cod and Potato Casserole

Serves 6 to 8

3 tablespoons extra virgin olive oil, plus more for greasing the baking dish

4 medium russet potatoes, peeled and thinly sliced on a mandoline, about $\frac{1}{16}$ inch thick

2 pounds cod fillets

2 sprigs of fresh rosemary, leaves picked and finely chopped (about $\frac{1}{4}$ cup)

Kosher salt and freshly ground pepper

This recipe requires a longer time in the oven, but the active time is minimal. You can prep everything before and assemble when you are ready to bake it. If you do that, keep the sliced potatoes in water in the fridge and pat them dry before layering them in the baking dish.

1. Preheat the oven to 375°F. Grease a 7 x 11-inch baking dish.
2. Place the potato slices in a large bowl and cover with cold water. Set aside for 10 minutes.
3. Rinse the fish under running water, then pat dry with paper towels.
4. Drain the potatoes, put them back in the same bowl, and pat them dry with a clean paper towel or a clean kitchen towel.
5. Add 2 tablespoons of the olive oil, half of the rosemary, and 2 generous pinches of salt and pepper to the bowl of potatoes and mix well to combine.
6. Layer the greased baking dish with about half of the potatoes, overlapping them. Add all of the fish to cover. Evenly add the remaining 1 tablespoon of olive oil over the fish, as well as a generous pinch of salt and the rest of the rosemary. Top with another layer of overlapping potatoes (you may have a few extra slices of potato left over).
7. Bake for 55 minutes, then turn the oven to broil and broil for an additional 3 to 4 minutes until the top browns (watch the broiler like a hawk, because things can go really wrong really fast with this level of high heat).

FRUITS

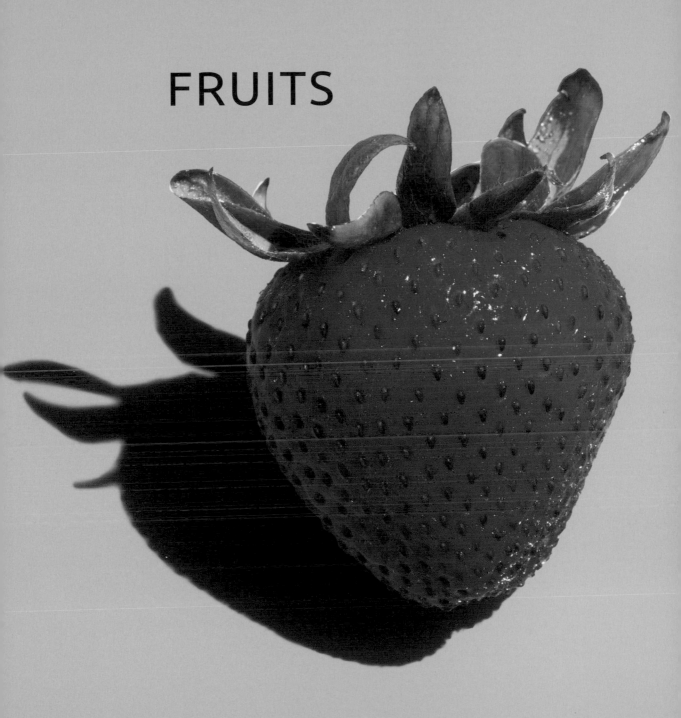

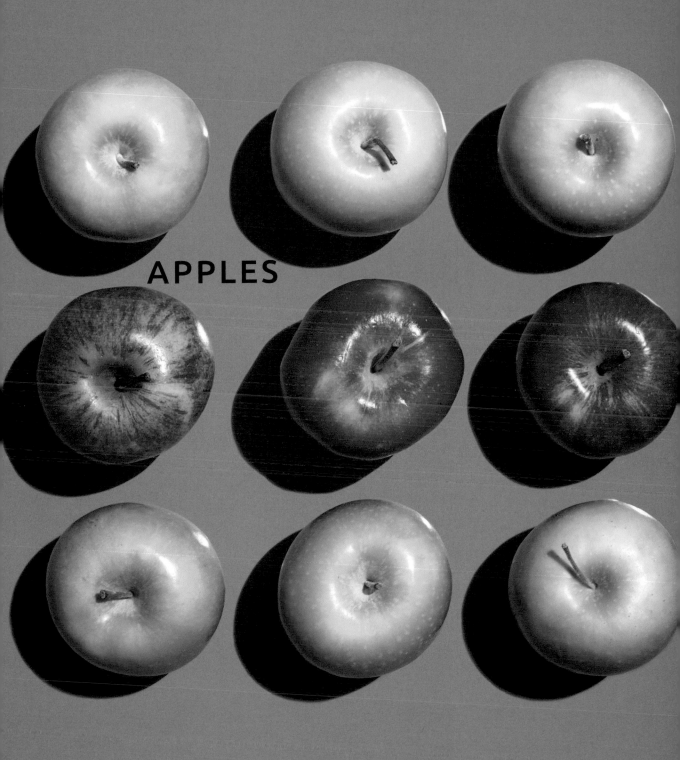

APPLES

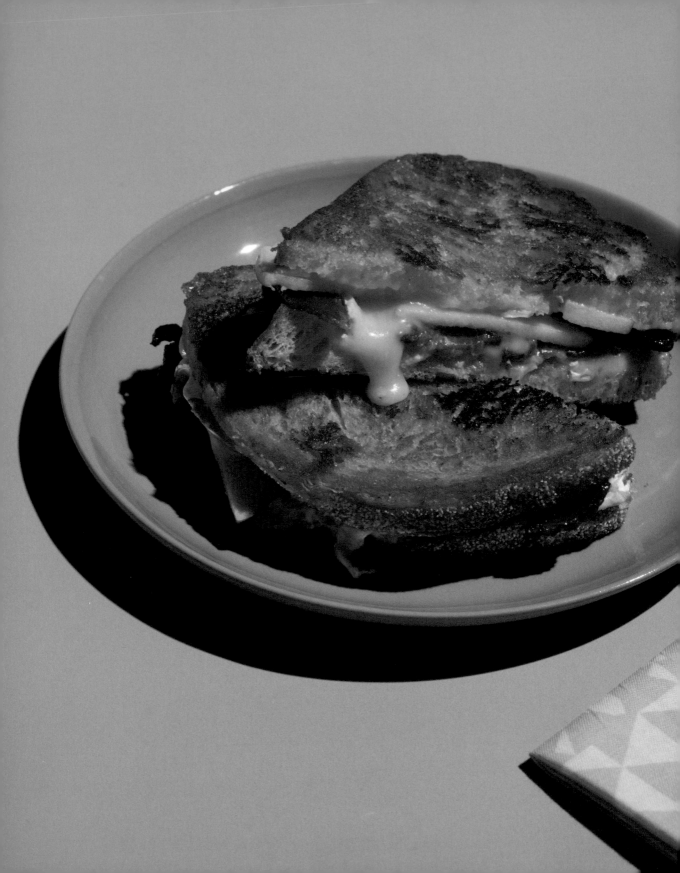

Apple Brie Bacon Grilled Cheese

Makes 4 sandwiches

At the time of recipe developing, we had to rock-paper-scissors for who got the last bites of this sandwich.

1. In a large skillet, cook the bacon over medium-high heat until crispy, about 4 minutes on both sides. Drain the bacon on paper towels, but reserve the bacon fat in the skillet.
2. Layer 4 slices of the bread with 2 slices of cheese, 4 slices of apple, 3 pieces of bacon, and 1 teaspoon of honey and finish with 2 more slices of cheese. Top each with a slice of bread.
3. Pour the bacon fat out of the skillet into a small bowl. Measure out 1 tablespoon of the bacon fat and return it to the skillet. Add 2 tablespoons of the butter and heat over high heat.
4. Place 2 of the sandwiches in the skillet and reduce the heat to medium-high. Cook for 4 minutes on each side, until the bread is browned and the cheese is fully melted. Remove the sandwiches from the skillet and set aside.
5. Add the remaining 2 tablespoons of butter and 1 tablespoon of bacon fat to cook the final 2 sandwiches in the same way. Serve immediately!

12 slices bacon
8 slices sourdough bread
1 (7-ounce) wheel camembert or brie cheese, cut into 16 slices
1 large Granny Smith apple, thinly sliced
4 teaspoons honey
4 tablespoons unsalted butter

Apple Slaw with Horseradish Vinaigrette

2 large Granny Smith apples,
   halved
4 carrots, peeled
2 celery stalks
½ bunch of fresh flat leaf parsley,
   leaves picked

DRESSING
2 tablespoons sour cream
2 tablespoons prepared
   horseradish
2 tablespoons maple syrup
2 tablespoons walnut oil
½ lemon, juiced
⅛ teaspoon cayenne pepper
Kosher salt and freshly ground
   black pepper

The crispy apples, carrots, and celery in this slaw are comple-mented by an unexpected kick from the horseradish and cayenne pepper, and the round flavors of the walnut oil.

1. Using a mandoline with the julienne attachment or with a knife, cut the apples and carrots into matchsticks. Thinly slice the celery. Place everything in a large bowl and sprinkle with the parsley.
2. Make the dressing: In a small bowl, whisk together the sour cream, horseradish, maple syrup, walnut oil, lemon juice, cayenne, and a pinch of salt and black pepper.
3. Add the dressing to the slaw and toss to combine. Taste and season with more salt and pepper.

Apple-Cranberry Galette

Serves 6 to 8

I learned how to make galettes recently and I absolutely love them because it doesn't matter how messy they look (it's called "rustic," OK?) and they never fail to impress. *Guest:* "You really made this whole thing from scratch?!" *Me:* "Oh this? Yeah, no big deal."

1. Preheat the oven to 375°F. Set aside a 15 x 10-inch baking sheet.
2. Make the dough: In a food processor, pulse the walnuts until they reach the consistency of bread crumbs. Add the spelt flour, granulated sugar, and a pinch of salt and pulse a few times to combine. Add the butter and process until the mixture looks like coarse meal. With the processor running, add the ice water 1 tablespoon at a time until the dough comes together and forms a ball. Remove the dough to a sheet of plastic wrap, form into a disk, wrap tightly, and store in the fridge for 30 minutes.
3. Make the filling: In a large bowl, add the apples, cranberries, orange zest, orange juice, brown sugar, cinnamon, all-purpose flour, and a pinch of salt. Toss to combine.
4. Remove the dough from the fridge and roll it out between 2 sheets of parchment paper to a 12-inch round. (If it's not a perfect round, that is totally OK, just be sure the rolled-out dough is roundish.) Carefully transfer to the baking sheet and remove the top layer of parchment paper.
5. Spoon the apple mixture into the center of the dough, leaving a 2-inch border all around. Fold the edges of the dough over to partially cover the apples.
6. Dot the filling with the butter cubes, distributing evenly.

DOUGH

½ cup walnuts

2 cups spelt flour

2 teaspoons granulated sugar

Kosher salt

¼ pound (1 stick) cold unsalted butter, cut into pieces

4 tablespoons ice water

FILLING

2 large Gala apples, peeled and sliced into thin wedges, about ¼ inch thick

1 cup frozen cranberries

1 orange, zested, ½ juiced

¼ cup packed light brown sugar

½ teaspoon ground cinnamon

1 tablespoon all-purpose flour

Kosher salt

1 tablespoon unsalted butter, cut into tiny cubes

TO FINISH

1 large egg

Granulated sugar, for sprinkling (optional)

Vanilla ice cream, for serving (optional)

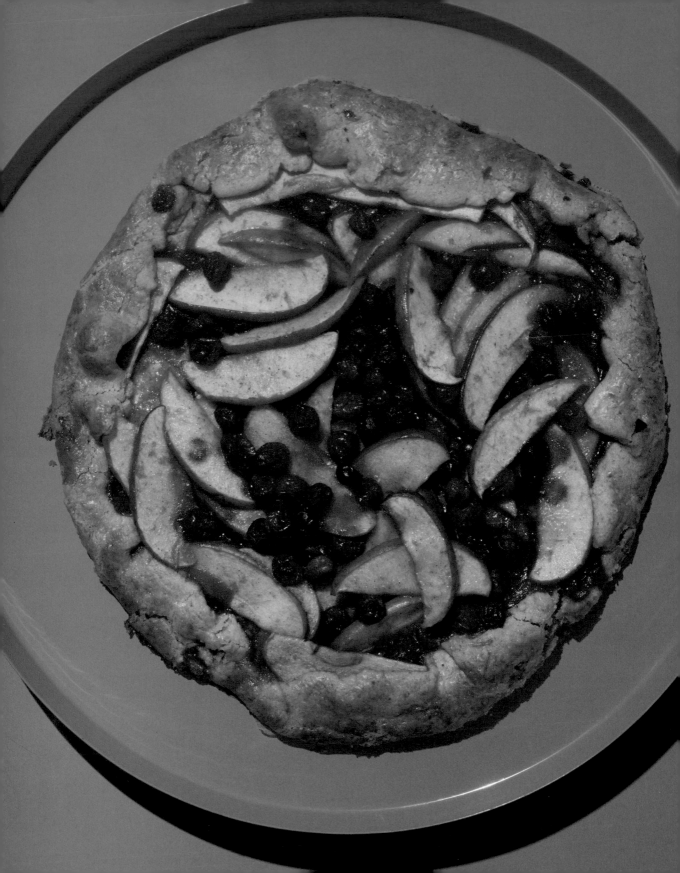

7. To finish: In a small bowl, whisk together the egg and 1 tablespoon water to make an egg wash. Brush the rim of the pastry with the egg wash and sprinkle with sugar (if using).
8. Bake until the dough is golden brown, about 45 minutes. Allow to cool before serving. Serve with vanilla ice cream, if desired.

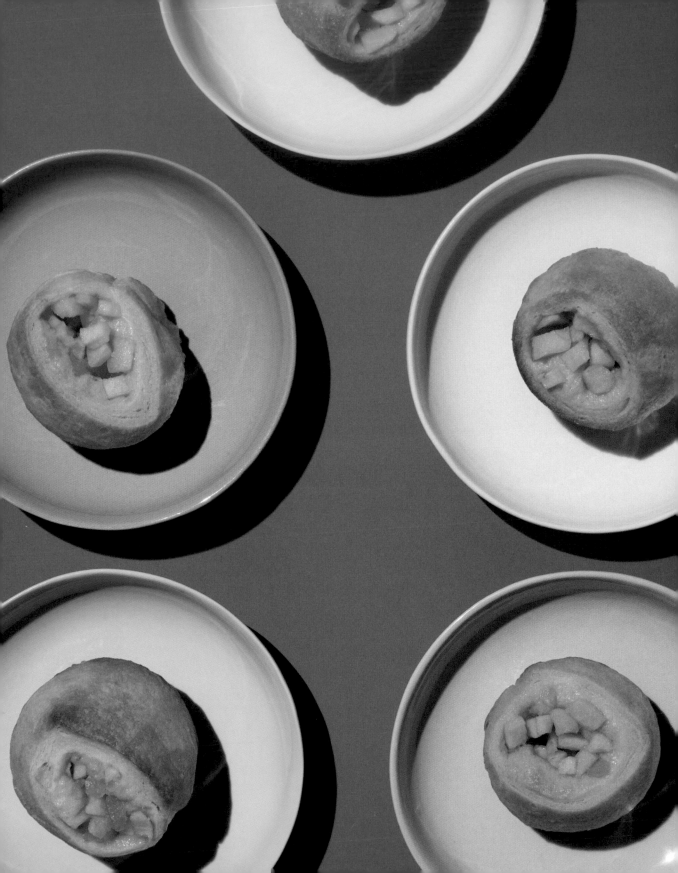

Apple-Ginger Cinnamon Rolls with a Grand Marnier Glaze

Makes 16 rolls

Making croissants or cinnamon rolls is not an impatient foodie–friendly endeavor. But by using some store-bought crescent roll dough, you can streamline a creative and delicious dessert. These would be delicious with vanilla ice cream and fresh whipped cream.

2 tablespoons unsalted butter, plus more for greasing the muffin tins
¼ cup finely chopped candied ginger
2 large Granny Smith apples, peeled, cored, and cut into ¼-inch cubes
¼ cup packed light brown sugar
Kosher salt
2 tablespoons granulated sugar
2 tablespoons ground cinnamon
2 (8-ounce) tubes crescent roll dough

GLAZE
½ cup powdered sugar
1 tablespoon Grand Marnier
1 orange, zested and juiced

1. Preheat the oven to 375°F.
2. In a medium saucepan, melt the 2 tablespoons of butter over low heat. Add the candied ginger and cook for 2 minutes.
3. Add the apples, brown sugar, and a pinch of salt to the pan. Stir well to combine, increase the heat to medium-high, and continue to stir frequently until the apples are soft, 5 to 8 minutes. Remove from the heat and allow to cool. IMPATIENT TIP: Place the apple mixture in the freezer to cool faster.
4. Butter 16 cups of 2 muffin tins and set aside.
5. In a small bowl, mix the granulated sugar and cinnamon.
6. Place a piece of parchment paper on a work surface. Remove the sheet of crescent roll dough from 1 tube and unroll it onto the parchment from left to right. Sprinkle the cinnamon-sugar evenly over the dough.
7. Scatter half of the apple mixture along the bottom of the dough, lengthwise. Using the parchment paper, roll the dough over the apple mixture going upward until you have a long log. Cut the log crosswise in half and cut each half into 4 equal pieces, giving you a total of 8 slices. Repeat with the remaining dough and apple mixture.
8. Place the slices in the buttered muffin cups. Bake until the rolls are golden, about 13 minutes.

9. Meanwhile, make the glaze: In a small bowl, whisk the powdered sugar, Grand Marnier, orange zest, and 2 tablespoons of the orange juice. Add more orange juice for a thinner glaze.

10. When the cinnamon rolls are done baking, allow them to cool slightly before glazing.

BANANAS

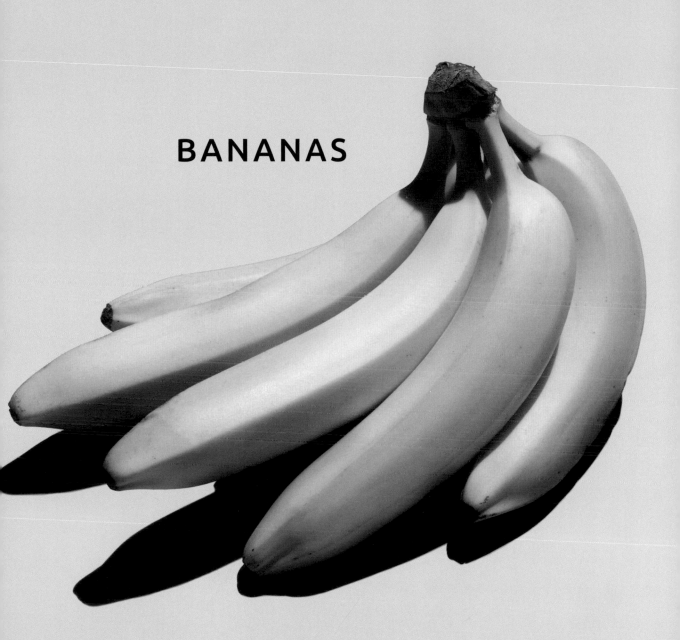

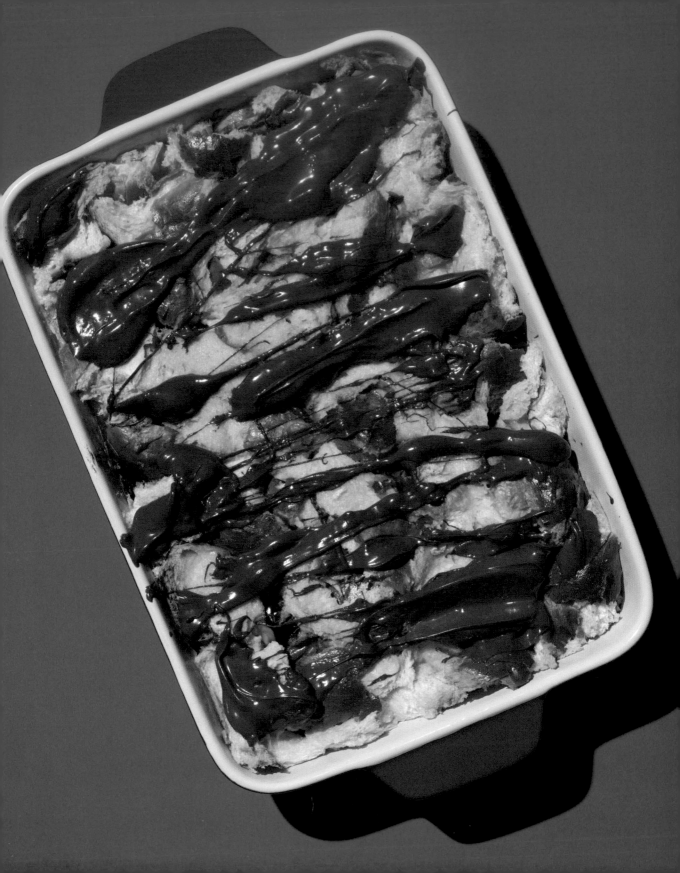

Chocolate Hazelnut Banana Bread Pudding

Serves 6 to 8

Confession: I REALLY hate bananas. I hate the way they look, the way they smell, the way they taste—Ewww! So naturally I decided to drown them in chocolate hazelnut spread and custard. I used Nocciolata, Rigoni di Asiago's palm oil–free chocolate hazelnut spread. If you can't find it at your local store, try Amazon or sub in another chocolate hazelnut spread. Now I love bananas (but only in this bread pudding).

Butter, for greasing the baking dish

1 loaf challah bread, torn into bite-size chunks

4 bananas, sliced

3 large eggs

1 cup heavy cream

2 cups whole milk

1 teaspoon vanilla extract

½ cup sugar

¼ teaspoon kosher salt

1 cup Nocciolata or chocolate hazelnut spread

Vanilla ice cream or whipped cream, for serving (optional)

1. Preheat the oven to 350°F. Butter a 7 x 11-inch baking dish.
2. Place half the challah in the bottom of the baking dish. Add the bananas, spreading them evenly around. Dollop ½ cup of the chocolate hazelnut spread over the bananas. Add the rest of the challah on top. Set aside.
3. In a large bowl, whisk the eggs, cream, milk, vanilla, sugar, and salt together. Pour the mixture over the challah and bananas.
4. Press the challah down with a spatula. Place parchment paper over the dish and place a weight on top. Let the bread soak for 30 minutes.
5. Cover the pudding with foil and bake for 30 minutes. Remove the foil and bake another 15 minutes. Allow to cool for 15 minutes.
6. While the pudding is cooling, place the remaining ½ cup of chocolate hazelnut spread in a small saucepan and heat over very low heat, stirring frequently, just until it runs off the spoon easily. Remove from the heat.
7. Drizzle the chocolate hazelnut spread over the pudding and serve immediately. This would be excellent with vanilla ice cream or whipped cream!

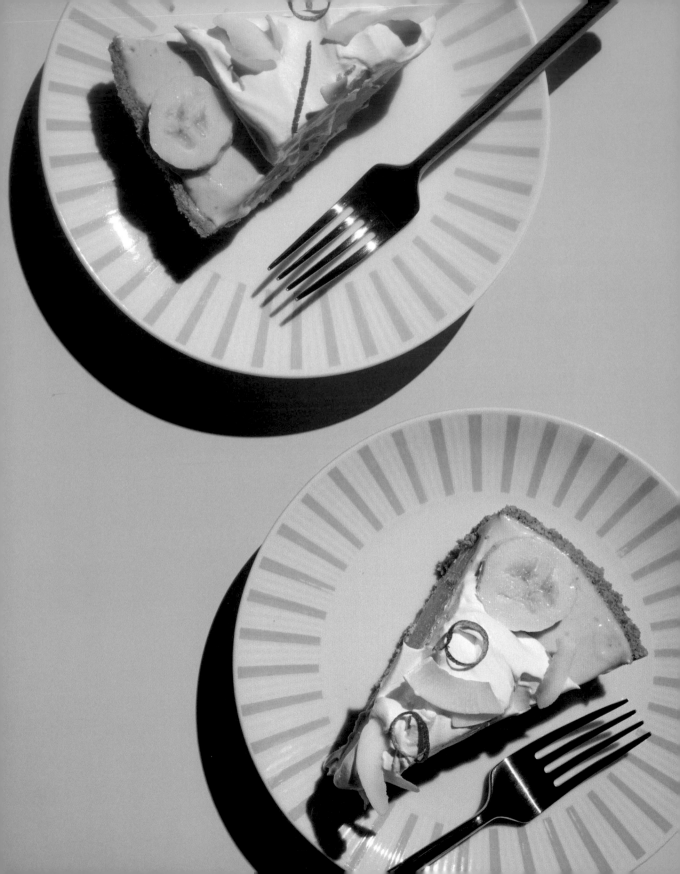

No-Bake Frozen Banana Pie

Serves 6 to 8

This no-bake pie is quick and easy to assemble and can be made ahead of time and stored in the freezer. Don't add the whipped cream topping until just before serving.

1. In a food processor, combine the bananas, powdered sugar, mascarpone, lime zest, and salt and process until smooth.
2. Pour the banana-mascarpone mixture into the graham cracker crust. Use the back of a spoon or an offset spatula to distribute the mixture evenly in the crust.
3. Freeze for a minimum of 2 hours or overnight.
4. For the topping: Toast the coconut flakes over medium-high heat in a small pan until the edges are slightly browned, 2 to 3 minutes. Stay vigilant because coconut flakes brown very quickly!
5. Remove the pie from the freezer and top it with the whipped cream. Add a sprinkle of the toasted coconut flakes and the sliced bananas. Slice and serve.

2 bananas, sliced
½ cup powdered sugar
16 ounces mascarpone cheese
Zest of 2 limes
⅛ teaspoon kosher salt
1 premade graham cracker crust

TOPPING
½ cup unsweetened coconut flakes
1 cup whipped cream
1 banana, sliced

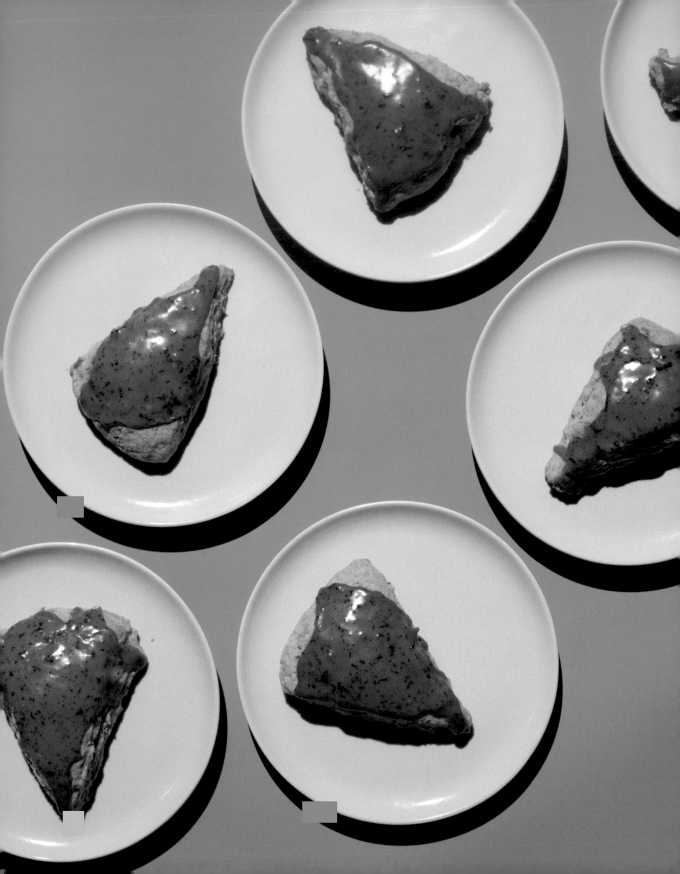

Banana Scones and Blueberry Glaze

Makes 10 to 14 scones, depending on how you portion them

Using a plain scone mix not only cuts down on ingredients and prep time, it also creates a good base layer to add in other flavors and bake a scone with a unique twist.

1. Preheat the oven to 425°F or according to the package directions. Line a 15 x 10-inch baking sheet with parchment paper.
2. In a bowl, mix the mashed banana, ½ cup of water, the cinnamon, and orange zest.
3. Make the scone dough according to the package directions, using the banana mixture to replace the water called for.
4. Form and bake the scones according to the package directions.
5. While the scones are baking, make the glaze: In a blender, puree the blueberries and powdered sugar on high speed until well combined, scraping the sides as necessary.
6. Remove the scones from the oven and cool slightly (about 5 minutes), then drizzle with the glaze and serve.

1 banana, mashed
½ teaspoon ground cinnamon
Zest of 1 orange
1 (14-ounce) box plain scone mix
Ingredients listed on the scone mix package for preparing the batter

BLUEBERRY GLAZE
¼ cup blueberries
1¼ cups powdered sugar

Banana Cardamom Oatmeal

Serves 4 to 6

1 (13.5-ounce) can unsweetened
    coconut milk

½ teaspoon ground cardamom

2 tablespoons honey

Kosher salt

2 cups extra-thick rolled oats

2 bananas, sliced

Maple syrup, for serving

½ cup raw pistachios, chopped, for
    garnish (optional)

Eating oatmeal every morning can get really boring really fast, am I right? This is an easy and delicious way to spice it up a bit. If you are just making it for yourself, you can make the whole recipe, store it in the fridge, and reheat with a little bit of water or milk for a quick "grab-n-go" breakfast for the week. Obviously, if you hate bananas like me, you can skip them.

1. In a medium saucepan, add the coconut milk, 1 cup of water, the cardamom, honey, and a pinch of salt. Whisk to combine over medium-high heat and bring to a boil.
2. As soon as the liquid is boiling, add the oats, reduce the heat to a simmer, and cook for 10 to 20 minutes, depending on the consistency you like.
3. Remove from the heat, add the bananas, and cover for 2 to 3 minutes.
4. Transfer to bowls and garnish each serving with a drizzle of maple syrup and top with chopped pistachios (if using).

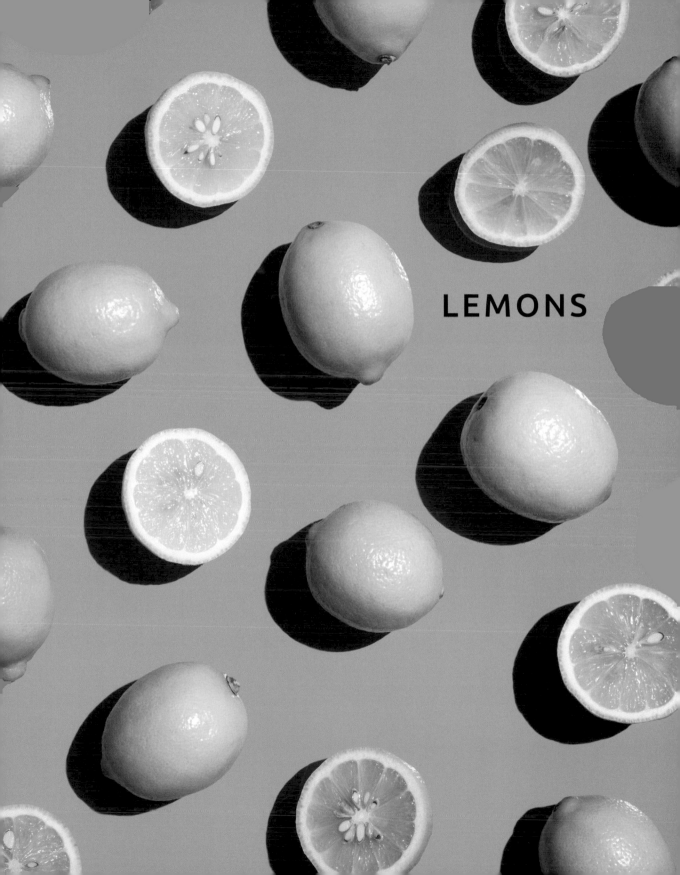

LEMONS

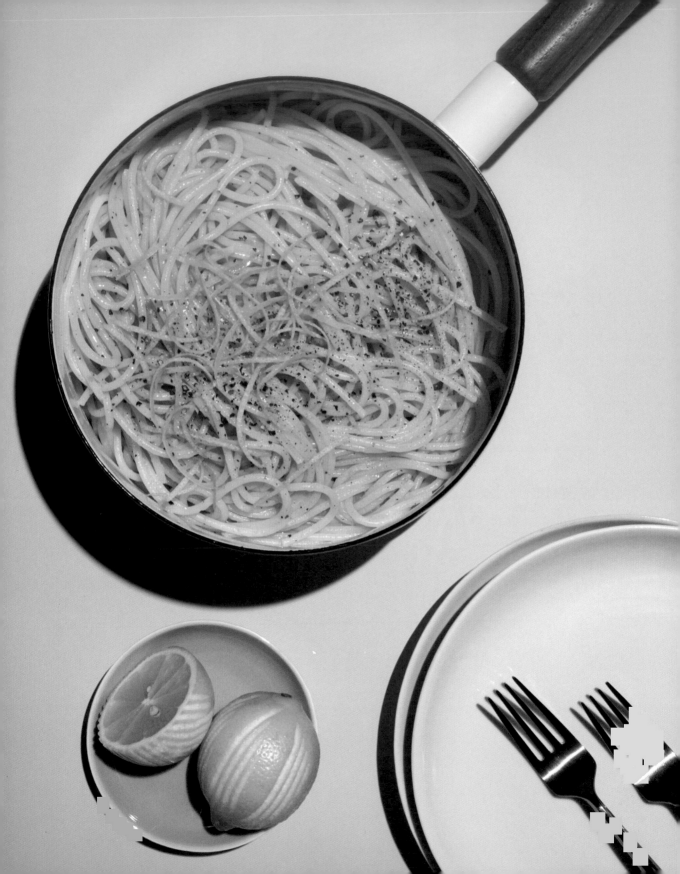

Uncle Robin's Lemon Spaghetti

Serves 4 to 6

I recently realized that the men on the mother's side of my family have invented some pretty genius recipes that are super fast and easy. Maybe my impatient foodie genes come from them? I mean, look, first there was my grandfather's spaghetti dish invention (see Rossellini Spaghetti on page 57) and now here is my uncle Robin's pasta made with just three main ingredients: Lemon, olive oil, and butter. I know it seems like a strange flavor combination that shouldn't really work, but I promise that it does.

Kosher salt
1 pound spaghetti or linguine
3 tablespoons extra virgin olive oil
1 lemon, zested and juiced
½ tablespoon unsalted butter, cut into small pieces
Freshly ground pepper
Fresh flat leaf parsley, chopped (optional)

1. Bring a large pot of salted water to a boil. Add the pasta and cook according to the package directions.
2. Meanwhile, in a small bowl, whisk together the olive oil and lemon zest. Taste and if you want a stronger lemon flavor, add the lemon juice, just 1 teaspoon at a time, until the desired flavor is reached.
3. Drain the pasta and transfer to a serving bowl. Top with the oil-lemon mixture, the butter, and a generous pinch of salt and pepper. Toss until well combined and the butter is completely melted. Top with parsley, if desired, and serve.

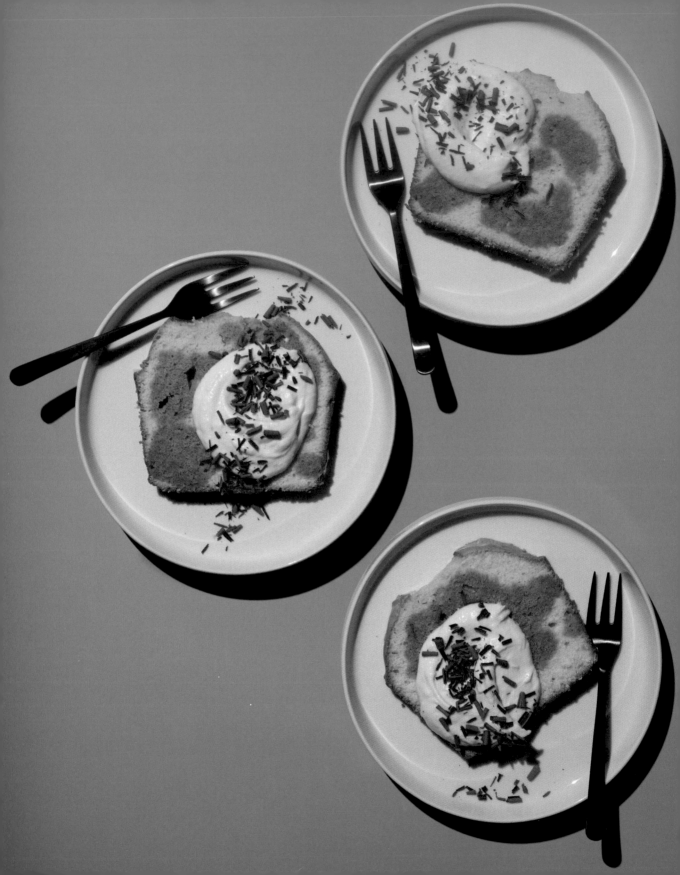

Deconstructed Impatient Tiramisu with Lemon-Mascarpone Cream

Serves 6 to 8

If I could fall asleep in gentle folds of this lemon-mascarpone cream, I would. If you can find a plain, premade pound cake, that will work too.

1. Preheat the oven to 350°F. Grease a 9 x 5-inch loaf pan. Set a piece of parchment paper inside so that pieces are hanging out the long sides of the loaf pan and grease the paper lightly.
2. Make the pound cake batter according to the package directions, then whisk in the lemon zest, lemon juice, and vanilla.
3. Pour the batter into the loaf pan and bake according to the package directions. Allow the cake to cool completely in the pan.
4. Meanwhile, make the lemon-mascarpone cream: With an electric hand mixer, whisk the egg whites until stiff peaks form, 2 to 3 minutes.
5. Rinse the mixer and, in a separate bowl, whisk the egg yolks with the sugar until light and creamy. Beat in the mascarpone and lemon zest. Using a silicone spatula, gently fold the egg whites into the mascarpone mixture. Store in the refrigerator until ready to serve.
6. To serve, place a ½-inch-thick slice of pound cake on a plate. Pour 1 to 2 tablespoons espresso over the cake. Add ¼ cup of the mascarpone cream and shave some dark chocolate on top. Enjoy!

POUND CAKE

Butter, coconut oil, or cooking spray, for greasing the pan
1 (16-ounce) box pound cake mix
Ingredients listed on the cake mix package for preparing the batter
2 lemons, zested and juiced
1 teaspoon vanilla extract

LEMON-MASCARPONE CREAM

3 large eggs, separated
¼ cup sugar
16 ounces mascarpone cheese
Zest of 3 lemons

FOR SERVING

1 cup espresso or strong coffee
A bar of your favorite dark chocolate

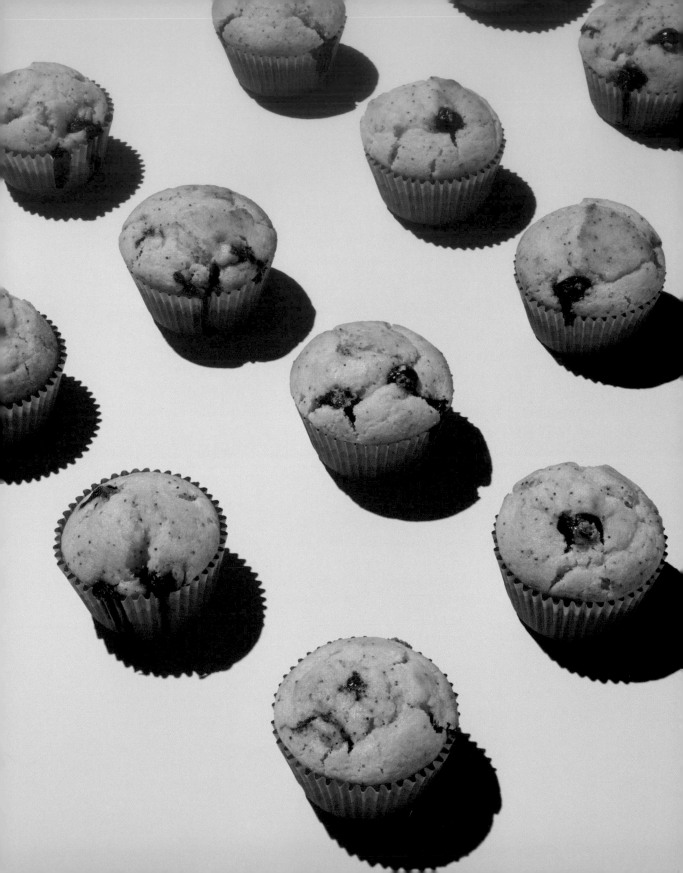

Lemon-Ricotta Poppy Seed Muffins

Makes 12 muffins

Fresh lemon zest, ricotta, and blueberries are a great way to elevate a simple muffin mix into something more interesting (and tasty).

1. Preheat the oven according to the muffin package directions. Coat 12 cups of a muffin tin with cooking spray or line with cupcake liners.
2. Make the muffin batter according to the package directions. Fold in the ricotta, lemon zest, poppy seeds, and blueberries.
3. Distribute the batter evenly among the muffin cups and bake for 20 minutes. Stick a toothpick or knife into the center of a muffin to see if it comes out clean. If it does, remove from the oven. If it doesn't, keep the muffins in the oven, checking at 5-minute intervals. Allow the muffins to cool in the pan before digging in.

Cooking spray, for greasing the muffin tins
1 (16-ounce) box cornmeal muffin mix
Ingredients listed on the muffin mix package for preparing the batter
½ cup ricotta cheese
Zest of 4 lemons
1 tablespoon poppy seeds
1 cup blueberries

Five-Ingredient Lemon Cookies

Makes about 15 cookies

1 large egg, lightly beaten
1 cup almond butter
½ cup sugar
Zest of 2 lemons
3 teaspoons raspberry or
  blueberry jam

When storing these cookies, make sure to keep them flat and to separate them with sheets of parchment, if you have to stack them. Otherwise jam will get all over the place!

1. Preheat the oven to 350°F. Line a 15 x 10-inch baking sheet with parchment paper.
2. In a medium bowl, add the egg, almond butter, sugar, and lemon zest. Mix until well combined.
3. Using a tablespoon, drop the dough onto the prepared baking sheet, spaced about 1 inch apart. Repeat until the dough is finished. Use the bottom of a teaspoon to make an indentation at the center of each cookie.
4. Bake until the dough starts to crack and brown, about 20 minutes. Remove from the oven and make the same indentations again.
5. Spoon ¼ teaspoon of the jam into each impression. Cool the cookies on a rack and serve.

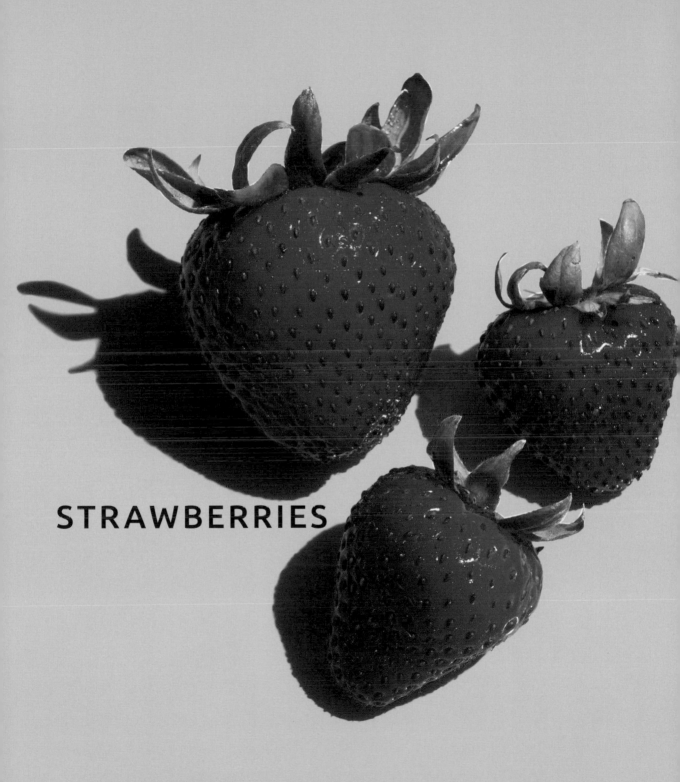

STRAWBERRIES

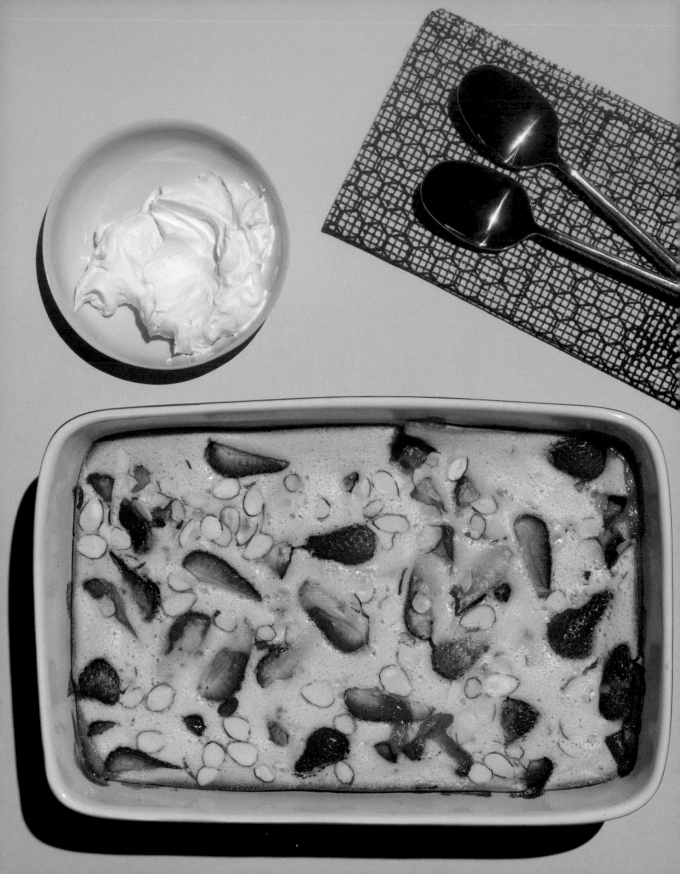

Spiced Strawberry Clafouti

Serves 6 to 8

Have you ever thought to yourself, "Can't I just dump some ingredients together without a lot of fuss and bake them and have an awesome cake come out?!" Well, please let me introduce you to the clafouti . . .

Butter, for greasing the baking
 dish
1 pound strawberries, quartered
1 cup all-purpose flour, plus more
 for flouring the baking dish
1 cup sugar
Kosher salt
2 large eggs
1 cup heavy cream
2 teaspoons almond extract
1 tablespoon grated fresh ginger
½ cup sliced almonds
Whipped cream (optional)

1. Preheat the oven to 350°F. Butter and lightly flour a 7 x 11-inch (2-quart) baking dish.
2. Scatter 3 cups of the strawberries in the baking dish and set aside.
3. In a large bowl, whisk together the flour, sugar, and a small pinch of salt. Create a little well in the center of the mixture.
4. Crack the eggs into the well and add the cream, almond extract, and ginger. Using a whisk or fork, beat the egg mixture into the flour mixture until it becomes a smooth batter.
5. Pour the batter over the strawberries. Place the remaining strawberries on top and scatter the sliced almonds evenly on top.
6. Allow the batter to rest for about 15 minutes before putting the baking dish in the oven (this will make your cake soft and tender and not chewy).
7. Bake until the dough is a light golden color, 25 to 30 minutes. Serve warm or at room temperature with or without whipped cream.

Strawberry and Rose Water Breakfast Oats

Serves 2

1 (13.5-ounce) can unsweetened
    coconut milk
2 cups sliced strawberries
2 tablespoons honey
1 teaspoon ground ginger
¼ teaspoon kosher salt
1 cup oats
¼ teaspoon rose water
¾ cup chopped raw pistachios

Another idea for how to bring a little excitement to morning oats. If strawberries and rose water aren't your thing, may I suggest our Banana Cardamom Oatmeal (page 180)?

1. In a blender, puree the coconut milk and 1 cup of the strawberries.
2. In a large saucepan, combine the strawberry-coconut milk with the honey, ginger, and salt and bring to a boil over medium-high heat.
3. Add the oats and stir to combine. Allow the mixture to return to a boil, then reduce the heat to a simmer, stir, and cover for 5 minutes. Set a timer—and no peeking!
4. When the timer goes off, stir in the remaining 1 cup of strawberries, cover, and cook another 3 to 5 minutes until the desired consistency of your oatmeal is achieved.
5. Remove from the heat, stir in the rose water and pistachios and serve.

Homemade Mini Strawberry Hand Pies

Makes 6 hand pies

I will forever feel equally affectionate about and traumatized by Pop-Tarts. In my early college years, eating Pop-Tarts for breakfast, lunch, snacks, and sometimes even dinner made me understand the saying "too much of a good thing." These little hand pies are my homage to my youth—a grown-up version (Grand Marnier icing!) of Pop-Tarts with way more flavorful and fresh ingredients.

1. Position a rack in the center of the oven and preheat the oven to 375°F. Line a 15 x 10-inch baking sheet with parchment paper.
2. Make the hand pies: In a small bowl, mix together the chopped strawberries, lime juice, honey, and flour. Set aside.
3. Unroll the pie dough carefully and use a 3½-inch round cutter (or drinking glass) to cut the dough into 12 rounds. Transfer the rounds to the lined baking sheet.
4. Spoon 1 tablespoon of the strawberry mixture in the center of 6 of the rounds. Place the other rounds on top and gently press a fork down to seal all the edges of the dough.
5. In a small bowl, whisk the egg and 1 tablespoon of water together to make an egg wash. Brush the pies with the egg wash and cut two tiny slits in the top of each pie.
6. Bake for 15 minutes, then rotate the baking sheet front to back, and bake until the dough is golden, another 10 minutes.
7. Meanwhile, make the icing: In a small bowl, whisk together the mashed strawberry, powdered sugar, and Grand Marnier.

HAND PIES

1 cup strawberries, finely chopped
½ lime, juiced
1 teaspoon honey
1 teaspoon all-purpose flour
2 store-bought refrigerated pie crusts (the rolled-up kind)
1 large egg

ICING

1 strawberry, mashed with a fork
1 cup powdered sugar
1 teaspoon Grand Marnier (or orange juice for kid-friendly hand pies)

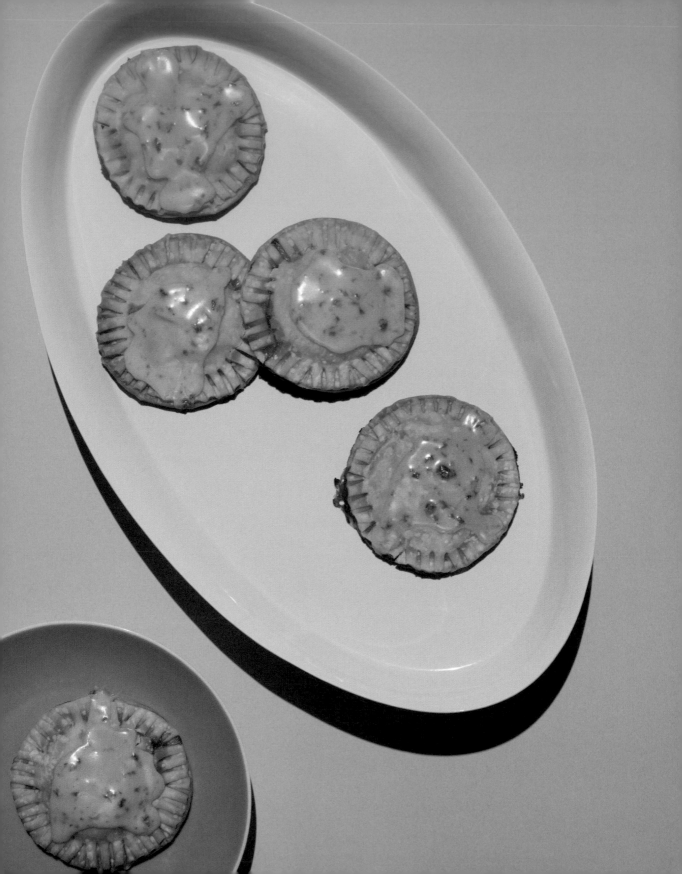

8. Remove the pies from the oven and allow to cool completely before icing. Once cooled, spoon about 1 tablespoon of icing over each pie and smooth with the back of a spoon. Enjoy!

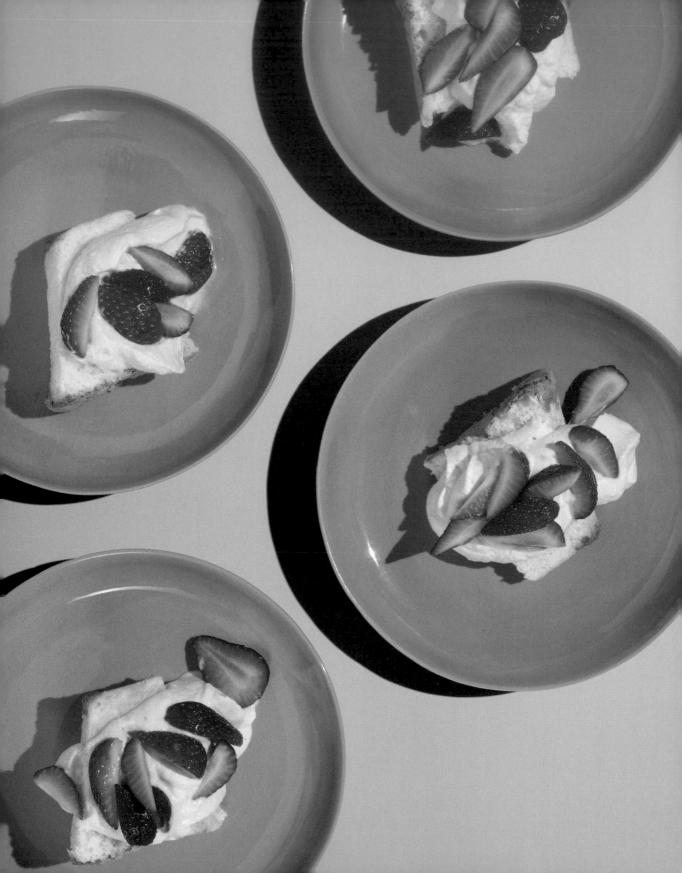

Aperol Spritz Cake

Serves 6 to 8

Since the early days of *Impatient Foodie*, Claudia, Davide, and I would often celebrate after a long day of cooking and shooting with an Aperol Spritz. This very impatient foodie–friendly cake is an ode to all the time, energy, and fun times we've shared bringing *Impatient Foodie* to life (including this cookbook!).

1 pound strawberries, sliced
1 cup sugar
2 cups heavy cream, chilled
1 vanilla bean, sliced open
     lengthwise
½ cup Aperol
1 orange, juiced
1 store-bought premade angel
     food cake
1 bottle Prosecco, chilled

1. In a medium bowl, combine the strawberries and ½ cup of the sugar. Cover with plastic wrap and set aside in the fridge.

2. Pour the heavy cream into a bowl and scrape the vanilla seeds into the cream. Using an electric hand mixer, whip the cream until soft peaks form, 5 to 7 minutes. Gradually pour in the remaining ½ cup of sugar, a bit at a time, whisking on high speed. Then slowly incorporate the Aperol and orange juice, whipping continuously. The cream can be slightly loose, if that is what you prefer.

3. To serve, slice the angel food cake into individual servings. Spoon about ¼ cup of the whipped cream over each slice. Pop the Prosecco and add ½ cup to the macerated strawberries and stir. Spoon the strawberry sauce over the whipped cream. Serve the rest of the Prosecco to drink with the dessert.

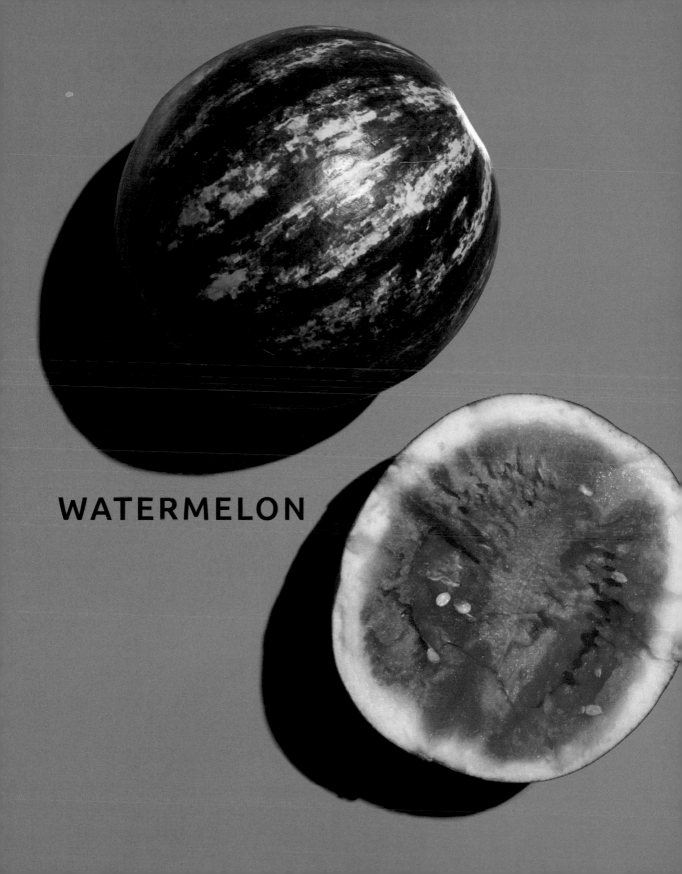

WATERMELON

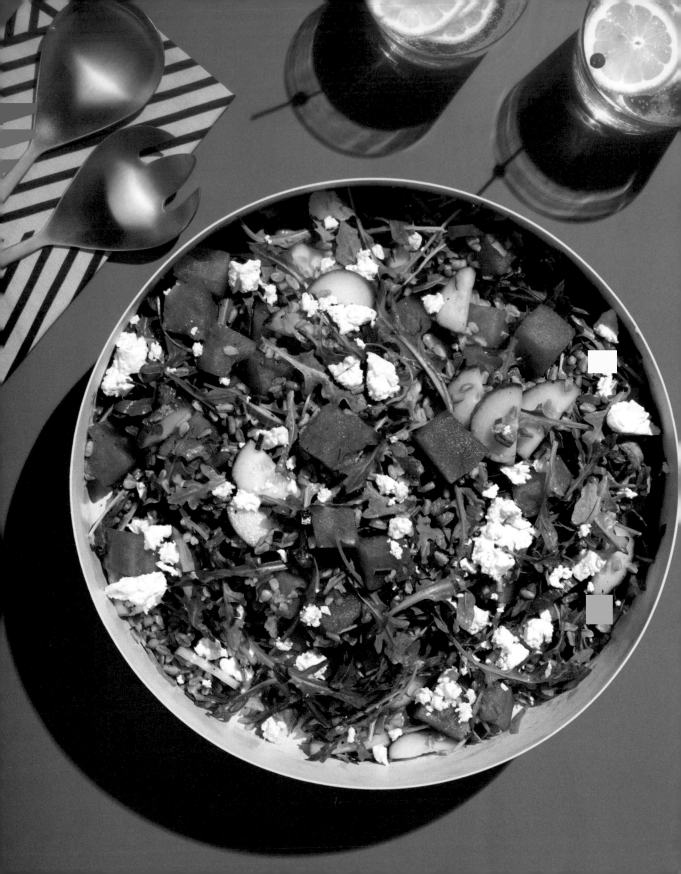

Farro Arugula Watermelon Salad

Serves 4 to 6

Watermelon is not often served in savory dishes, but this salad really works and is perfect on a hot summer's day.

1. Cook the farro according to the package directions.
2. Meanwhile, in a large salad bowl, whisk together the olive oil, lime juice, and salt and pepper to taste.
3. When the farro is done cooking and slightly cooled, add it to the salad bowl and gently toss with the vinaigrette. Add the red onion, cucumber, and arugula and toss gently to combine with the farro. Top with the watermelon and feta. Drizzle with balsamic glaze and serve.

1 (8.8-ounce) package farro
⅓ cup extra virgin olive oil
1 lime, juiced
Kosher salt and freshly ground pepper
1 small red onion, finely chopped
1 English (seedless) cucumber, halved lengthwise and sliced into half-moons
1 (5-ounce) container prewashed arugula
3 cups bite-size pieces watermelon, rind and seeds removed
4 ounces feta cheese, crumbled
1 teaspoon balsamic glaze

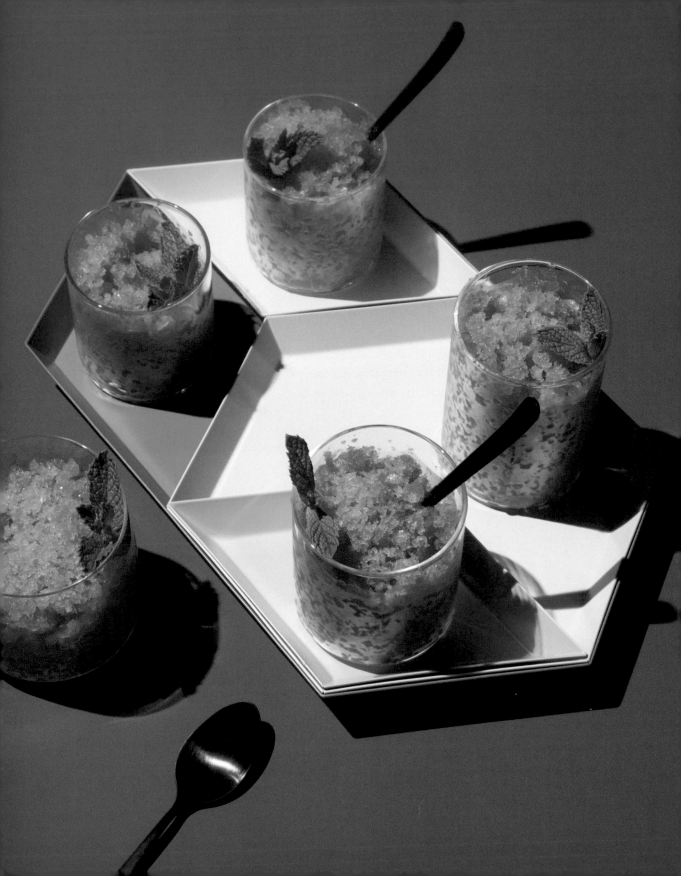

Watermelon Granita with Peaches, Lime, and Mint Garnish

Serves 6 to 8

This recipe requires some planning ahead as it has to freeze through before you serve it. It's important to occasionally open up the freezer and scrape the mixture with a fork—a strangely satisfying sensation.

8 cups roughly chopped
    watermelon, rind and seeds
    removed
2 peaches, peeled and coarsely
    chopped
2 limes, juiced
½ cup sugar
Fresh mint leaves, for garnish

1. In a blender, combine the watermelon, peaches, lime juice, and sugar and blend until liquefied. Pour into a shallow baking dish and place in the freezer. Set a timer for 2 hours.
2. When the timer goes off, scrape the mixture with a fork, especially along the sides of the pan. Freeze for another 2 to 3 hours, scraping the granita once every hour.
3. To serve, spoon the granita into a serving bowl or a glass. Garnish with mint leaves.

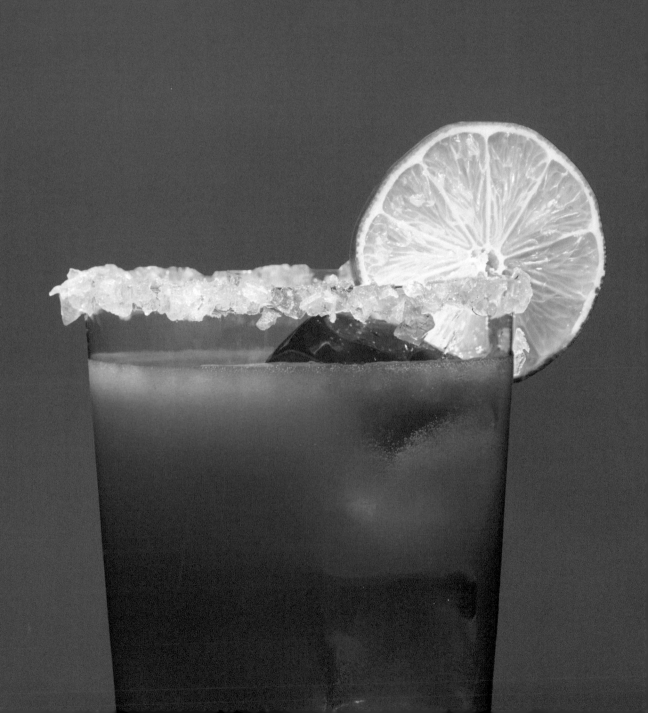

Watermelon Jolly Rancher Margarita

Makes 1 cocktail

The fact that this cocktail tastes like a watermelon Jolly Rancher was not intentional, but very welcomed.

1. Pour 2 tablespoons of agave into a saucer and 2 tablespoons of the Maldon salt into a separate saucer. Dip the rim of a glass in the agave and then in the salt to coat.
2. In a cocktail shaker, muddle the watermelon, jalapeño, and ½ ounce of agave nectar together. Add the lime juice, tequila, and ice and shake. Strain over fresh ice in the rimmed glass. Garnish with lime or jalapeño.

½ ounce agave nectar, plus 2 tablespoons for rimming the glass
Maldon salt
2 (1-inch) cubes watermelon, rind and seeds removed
2 slices jalapeño pepper, ribs removed and seeded
1 ounce fresh lime juice
2 ounces blanco tequila
1 lime wheel or jalapeño slice, for garnish

Watermelon Chia Breakfast Pudding

Serves 4 to 6

1 cup full-fat Greek yogurt
1 cup raw coconut water
¼ cup chia seeds
1½ cups ½-inch cubes
  watermelon, rind and seeds
  removed (reserve ½ cup for
  garnish)
½ cup strawberry jam
Granola
1 cup sliced strawberries, for
  garnish
Topping options: Honey, maple
  syrup, bee pollen, or whatever
  you desire

Chia pudding always takes some time to set, so it's not entirely impatient friendly. The good thing about it, though, is that you can make it in bulk to have a prepared, fast-grab breakfast for the week. The active time for this recipe is about ten minutes. Then you stick it in the fridge and forget about it for a few hours while it does its thing and thickens up into a delicious pudding.

1. In a small bowl, combine the yogurt, coconut water, and chia seeds. Store in the fridge and allow to thicken for about 1 hour.
2. Meanwhile, in a blender, combine 1 cup of the watermelon cubes and the jam and pulse until just combined. Set aside.
3. When ready to serve, layer the yogurt-chia mixture, watermelon-strawberry jam, and some granola in a glass or bowl. Top with sliced strawberries and the reserved watermelon cubes. Add additional toppings of your choice and enjoy.

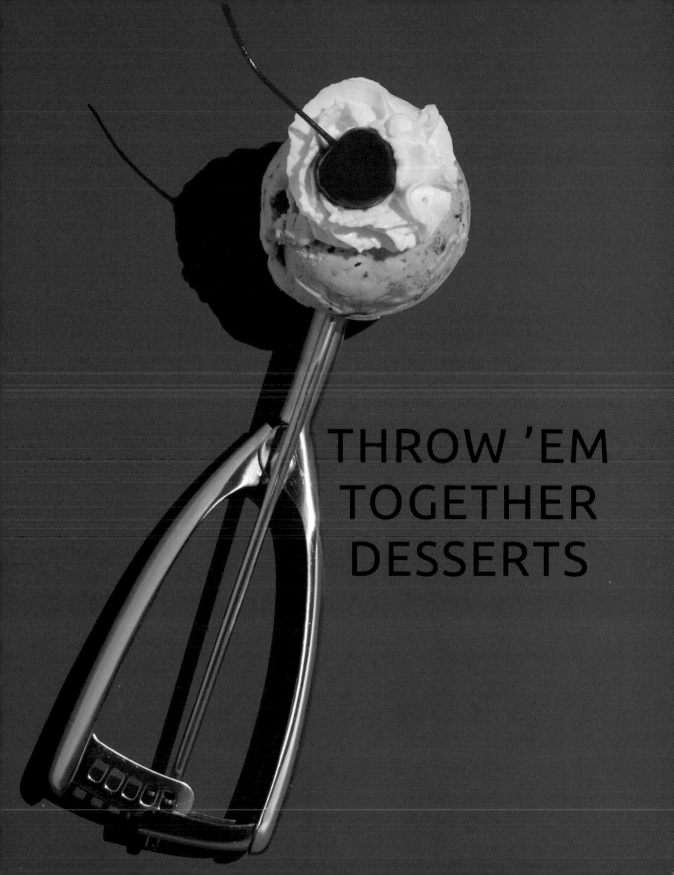

THROW 'EM
TOGETHER
DESSERTS

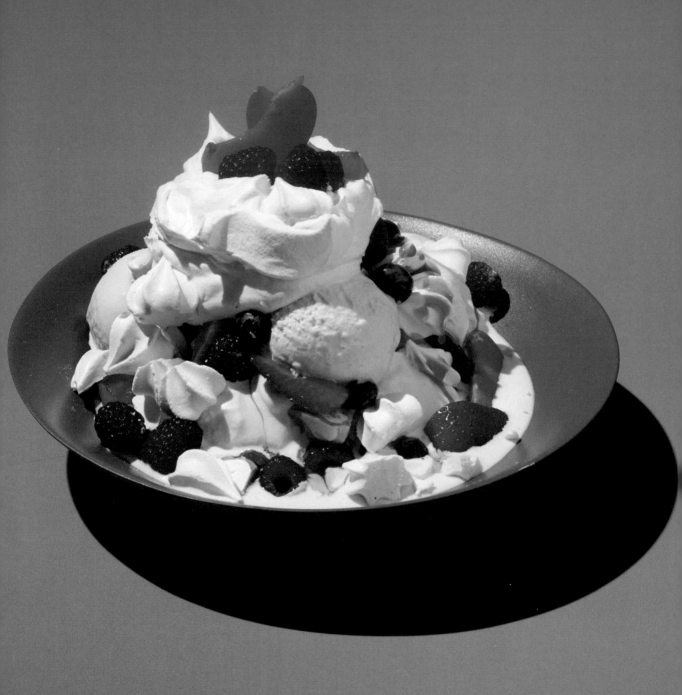

Lotte's Mess

Serves 4 to 6

Credit for this version of Eton mess goes to a young lady I had dinner with in Sweden a few summers ago. Lotte works long hours as a baker in the summers, and I loved that she came up with a dessert that required minimal time and no baking. This is an ideal dessert for a dinner party because you can assemble at the last minute. Just be sure to take your ice cream out of the freezer while people are enjoying their main course to allow it to soften sufficiently.

1 pint vanilla ice cream, slightly softened
2 cups roughly chopped mini meringues
½ cup chocolate sauce
½ cup caramel sauce
Whipped cream
Berries in season

In a large bowl, combine the ice cream and meringues, using a large spoon to mix well. Drizzle the chocolate sauce and caramel sauce over everything, followed by a slightly obscene amount of whipped cream and finally the berries. Serve immediately.

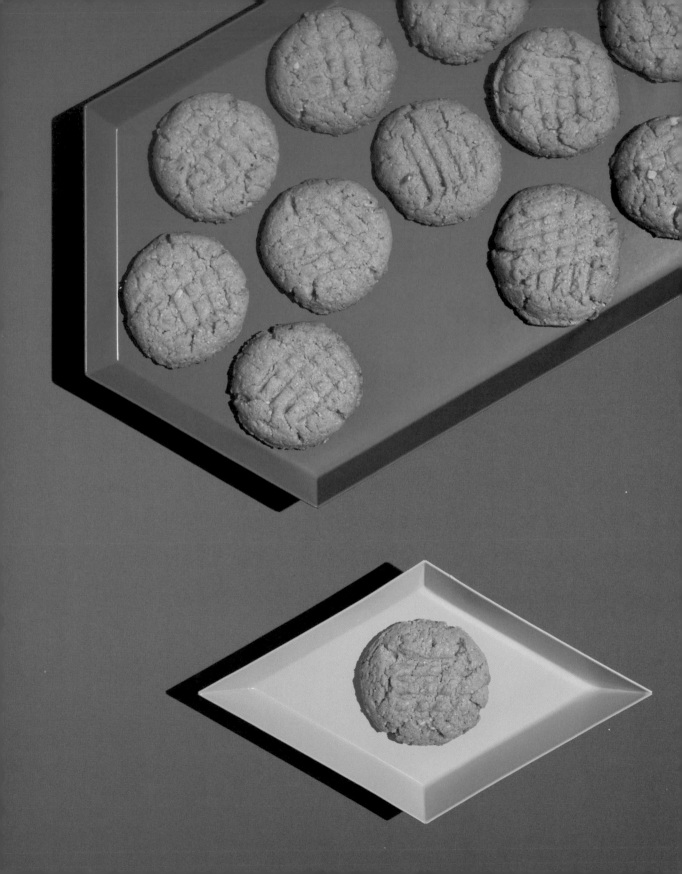

Orange Blossom Cashew Butter Cookies with Star Anise

Makes about 16 cookies

Cashew butter can be expensive, but Trader Joe's has some decently priced options.

1 large egg
1 cup cashew butter
½ cup sugar
½ teaspoon orange blossom water
Kosher salt
1 star anise
canola oil, for greasing two spoons

1. Preheat the oven to 350°F. Line a 15 x 10-inch baking sheet with parchment paper.
2. In a large bowl, lightly beat the egg. Add the cashew butter, sugar, orange blossom water, and a small pinch of salt and mix until well combined. Using a fine grater, grate 3 arms of the star anise into the bowl and stir to combine.
3. Grease 2 spoons—one tablespoon and one teaspoon—with canola oil. Use the tablespoon to scoop the dough, then drop the dough onto the prepared baking sheets, spacing them about 1 inch apart. The other spoon can come in handy if things get sticky.
4. Dip a fork in a glass of warm water and make a crosshatch design into the top of the cookies.
5. Bake until the cookies are golden brown and the dough just begins to crack, 12 to 15 minutes. Transfer the cookies on the parchment to a rack and allow to cool slightly before serving.

Brownie Ice Cream Cake

Serves 6 to 8

If you've always thought of ice cream cakes as territory of professionals with lots of patience, this brownie ice cream cake will change your mind.

Butter, for greasing the pan
1 (18.4-ounce) box brownie mix
Ingredients listed on brownie mix box for preparing the batter
1 pint strawberry ice cream
1 (12-ounce) jar raspberry jam
1 pint vanilla ice cream
1 (16-ounce) container Cool Whip, thawed
2 cups raspberries or blueberries (or both!)

1. Preheat the oven according to the brownie package directions. Line the bottom of a 12 x 17-inch rimmed baking sheet with parchment paper. Butter the parchment paper and the sides of the pan.
2. Make the brownie batter according to the package directions. Spread the batter onto the baking sheet and bake for 15 minutes.
3. Meanwhile, remove the ice cream from the freezer and place in the fridge to soften.
4. Cool the brownies to room temperature. Cut the brownies into three 9 x 5-inch rectangles (use the bottom of the loaf pan as a guide).
5. Line all sides of a 9 x 5-inch loaf pan with plastic wrap, ensuring that there is excess wrap hanging over the sides. This will be used to layer the cake.
6. Layer the cake in the prepared pan in the following order: A layer of brownie, a layer of strawberry ice cream using half of the ice cream, a thin layer of raspberry jam, a layer of brownie, a layer of vanilla ice cream using all of the ice cream, a layer of raspberry jam, the last brownie, and a layer of the remaining strawberry ice cream. Wrap the ends of the plastic wrap over the top of the loaf pan and gently push down on the cake to pack the layers tightly. Freeze for a minimum of 3 hours, or overnight.
7. To serve, place a plate upside down on top of the loaf pan

and flip over to remove the cake, gently pulling on the plastic wrap to help.

8. Coat the entire cake in a thick layer of Cool Whip, spreading it evenly with a spatula. Decorate with fresh raspberries and blueberries and enjoy!

ACKNOWLEDGMENTS

I have to start off my acknowledgments with a few people who jumped on to the *Impatient Foodie* bandwagon from the get-go and encouraged me to keep going, even through the moments where I felt like having a food blog was the most pointless/stupid thing ever: Davide Luciano, Claudia Ficca, and Noah Stein—I adore you all, thank you for everything you have done. I also want to thank my manager, Hilla Narov, for all her support and advice over the years. There have been many times when I felt totally lost in what to do and how to do it and Hilla was there to help me map out next steps and stay plowing (strategically) ahead. Hilla makes me do mind maps every few months, but I love her anyway. Thank you to my parents, who have been incredible role models for me my whole life and are wonderful, loving, fun, positive human beings—I love you so much and am so grateful for you and to you. As I have been reviewing this book and my blog, I realized I talk a lot about my dad, my grandad, and various other family members, but not much love spread to my "dear old mamma," so I want to remedy that here: My mom is an absolute inspiration to me and is someone whom I admire and love hugely. She also taught me all the basics about cooking, which gave me the foundational skills I needed to figure out my own flair. I'd never be in the kitchen if it weren't for her early cooking lessons and guidance. Grazie mamma! To my dearest, closest friends who have shared my *Impatient Foodie* posts and suffered through multiple tastings—you know who you are and I love you. A huge thank-you to Caleb Lane, who ate all ninety-eight recipes in this cookbook and provided honest notes, and helped me get through the cookbook-writing process without any trips to the crazy house—*Ti amo*. Thank you to Christene Barberich, who has taught me so much and been an incredible loving, patient, encouraging mentor. So much of my writing, thinking, and perspective have also been shaped by my dear friend Mikki Halpin—thank you for all your words of wisdom and guidance. Thank you also to Alex Brannian, Allison Foley, Lara Backmender, Tom Cinko, Brian von Glahn, and Cindy Gasparre. I am also incredibly grateful for people directly responsible for making this cookbook a reality, my book agents, David Kuhn and Laura Nolan, and the Scribner team: Shannon Welch, Nan Graham, Roz Lippel, Jessica Yu, John Glynn, Kara Watson, Ashley Gilliam, and Jaya Miceli—thank you infinitely for all your encouragement, help, and support.

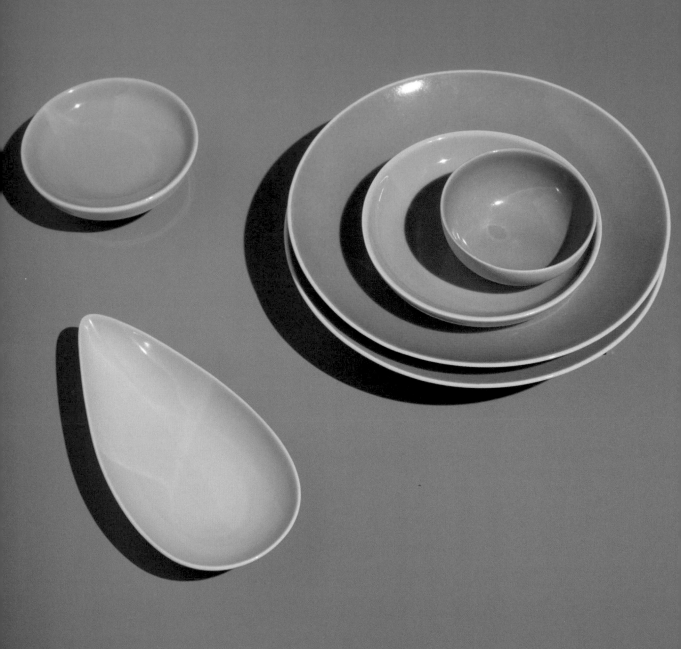

INDEX